Laboratory Manual to Accompany

ASSEMBLING AND REPAIRING PERSONAL COMPUTERS

Second Edition

Dan L. Beeson

Prentice Hall
Upper Saddle River, New Jersey Columbus, Ohio

Pearson Education
Upper Saddle River, New Jersey 07458

Printed in the United States of America

10 9 8 7 6 5 4 3 2 1

ISBN: 0-13-086111-1

This manual is to accompany ASSEMBLING AND REPAIRING PERSONAL COMPUTERS by Dan Beeson. The corresponding chapters in the text should be read before doing any laboratory, and the text should be kept handy as a reference guide.

Because of the wide range of differing equipment each facility will have, and the need in many cases for specific documentation, labs are generic. Instructor preparation before and guidance during the lab are crucial.

TABLE OF CONTENTS

EQUIPMENT REQUIRED FOR THESE LABS

Functioning system consisting of at least:

- case and power supply
- motherboard with cpu and ram (386up & 2 Meg for Windows)
- keyboard (and a bad keyboard for stripe repair and soldering)
- display (and matching video adapter card)
- 3 1/2" floppy drive (and matching controller card)
- 5 1/4" floppy drive (")
- hard drive (")
- DOS installed on hard drive

Support Equipment

- variable lab power supply (dual if possible)
- DOS to install
- Windows to install
- printer cable
- paper for printer
- parallel printer (dot matrix, possibly ink jet and laser)
- parallel & serial loopback connectors
- mouse, bus mouse adapter card or serial card (or unused port)
- mouse software
- resistor color code chart
- resistors : 47 Ω, 1 KΩ, 2.2 KΩ, 47 KΩ, 330 KΩ
- power supply load resistor packs (22ohm/2watt or see text)
- analog and/or digital multimeter
- complete soldering kit with diag cutters, hobby knife, wick
- alternate displays with matching controllers
- alternate floppy drives with matching controllers
- alternate hard drives with matching controllers
- post diagnostic add in card with documentation
- box of "bad" motherboards
- box of "bad" keyboards
- diskette with "bad" fat table
- tape backup drive with driver software and FORMATTED tape
- sound card, driver software, speakers, microphone
- system with Windows, diskette with .wav files
- sound card test program
- CD-ROM drive with controller (possibly on sound card)
- CD-ROM driver software, and CDs
- soldering kit (if facilities permit)
- Fax/modem kit with software
- Optical scanner controller card, optical scanner, driver software

Toolkit containing at least:

- #1 & #2 phillips screwdriver
- 1/4" nut driver
- anti-static wriststrap
- chip puller

Bootable DOS disk(s) containing at least:

- attrib
- backup or MSbackup
- chkdsk
- command.com
- defrag
- debug
- fdisk
- format
- memmaker
- mem
- msd
- recover
- restore (or MSbackup)
- scandisk

Bootable disk containing your preferred diagnostic program(s)

- (qaplus, checkit, or amidiags, the troubleshooter, or similar programs)
- low level format programs (if instructor desires)

1 INTRODUCTION LAB

PURPOSE: To give student initial familiarization with components inside the system they will be using for this course.

EQUIPMENT:

Functioning system
bootable DOS floppy, should have at least:
chkdsk, mem

toolkit, should contain at least :
- #2 phillips screwdriver
- 1/4" nut driver
- anti-static wrist strap

PROCEDURE:

1. Examine the outside of the system and identify the system makeup. Plug the display signal cable into the matching jack on the rear of the system. Plug the display power cable into power. Plug the keyboard into the matching jack on the rear of the system. Plug the system power cable into the matching jack on the rear of the system (on the power supply). If you have a mouse, insert the plug in the matching jack.

2. If you have NO hard drive, insert a bootable DOS floppy in floppy drive A:. Turn on display power. A COLD boot is turning on the system power. Boot the system to see that it works! The system first performs a Power On Self Test (POST). You should :

a. hear or feel the fan begin
b. see keyboard LEDs flash from power up
c. hear the hard drive wind up and spin
d. see video card ROM message on screen
e. see system ROM BIOS header on screen
f. hear the POST RAM memory test and see it on the display
g. see keyboard LEDs flash from POST
h. see drive A: LED and hear head seek
i. see drive B: LED and hear head seek
j. see hard drive C: LED
k hear one beep of POST confirming all OK
l. see system ROM BIOS configuration message on display
(usually showing installed equipment and memory)
m. booting from hard drive
n see a starting MS-DOS message

o. see a few messages from the config.sys file
p. see a few messages from the autoexec.bat file
q. see a C:\> prompt if you have a hard drive or
see an A:\> if you have a bootable floppy in drive A:

Examine the BIOS display and copy the information down. If it is scrolled up off the screen too quickly, us the PAUSE key to stop the display, and the RETURN to continue when done. Type the command "DIR". The system should show the files on the disk. If it does this, continue. If NOT, or if you hear a series of beeps (audio error codes) or see an error warning and number on the screen (video error code), consult the instructor.

3. The cover is usually held on by 6 to 8 screws in the back. **Turn the system off** (display also), and remove the cover carefully. Examine the inside, identifying parts. Before you touch any parts, use static control procedures explained by your instructor, including using an anti-static wrist strap connected to a bare steel area of the system case.

4. Fill in the chart below.
(Instructor guidance required, Instructions follow list.)

A. Processor type and speed __________

B. Type and amount of memory __________
DIP or SIMM

C. Floppy drives installed __________
3 1/2" and/or 5 1/4"

D. Hard drives installed __________
Model usually labeled

E. Video adapter and display __________
label on rear of display

F. Peripherals or Ports installed __________

G. I/O expansion slot type (8bit ISA,
16 bit ISA,Vesa, Eisa) __________

H. Presence and size of cache __________

I. Brand of Rom Bios __________

5. Replace the cover, turn on system to verify that it still works.

To determine the answers above, refer to instructors directions and the list below:

A. The processor is either a 40 pin dip or a SMT (Surface Mount Technology) chip looking like a small square black cracker with over 100 leads. The Type and speed is typed on top. The type will probably be an 8088, 80286, 80386, or 80486. Speeds will be 10, 12, 16, 25, 33, 40, 50, or 66 Megahertz.

B. Most systems do a memory check on booting during the POST. Note this value. To physically check, locate the memory banks inside. If in dips, with 4 banks of 9 chips, read the number on top of the chip. In a few instances the number will be undecipherable, and you must look at manufacturers specifications. If in SIPs or SIMMs (which are little printed circuit boards with their own chips on them), examine the chips on each bank. You may try the DOS command MEM to see memory usage. The command CD\DOS may be required first to tell the computer where the program is.

C. Floppy drives are visible from the front of the system. The physical size is either 5 1/4 inch or 3 1/2 inch. The density is NOT always easily physically identifiable. Entering the SETUP program will show what the machine THINKS it has. Doing a DIRectory command with a high density diskette installed will prove if it can read the high density or not. Floppies are usually drive A: or B:, so DIR A: and DIR B: should show a directory of the floppy in each drive.

D. Hard drives may NOT be visible from the outside. Manufacturer part number may be used to look up the specifications. You may try the DOS command CHKDSK to see drive sizes. (Scandisk is not as quick for this glance at drives.)

E. The video adapter card will have crystals of certain speeds, and a certain amount of memory. The pin out (see text chapter on displays) of the signal cable from the display will narrow the identification of the display to mono/cga/ega (9pins) or vga/supervga (15 pins modified D shell [possible pin locations on plug, may not all be used]).

F Peripherals and ports are detailed in the text chapter on peripherals. A 25 or 9 pin male D shell is a serial port. A 25 pin female D shell is a parallel port. A 15 pin female standard sized D shell is a game port.

G. See Figure below or text chapter on motherboard, chapter on busses.

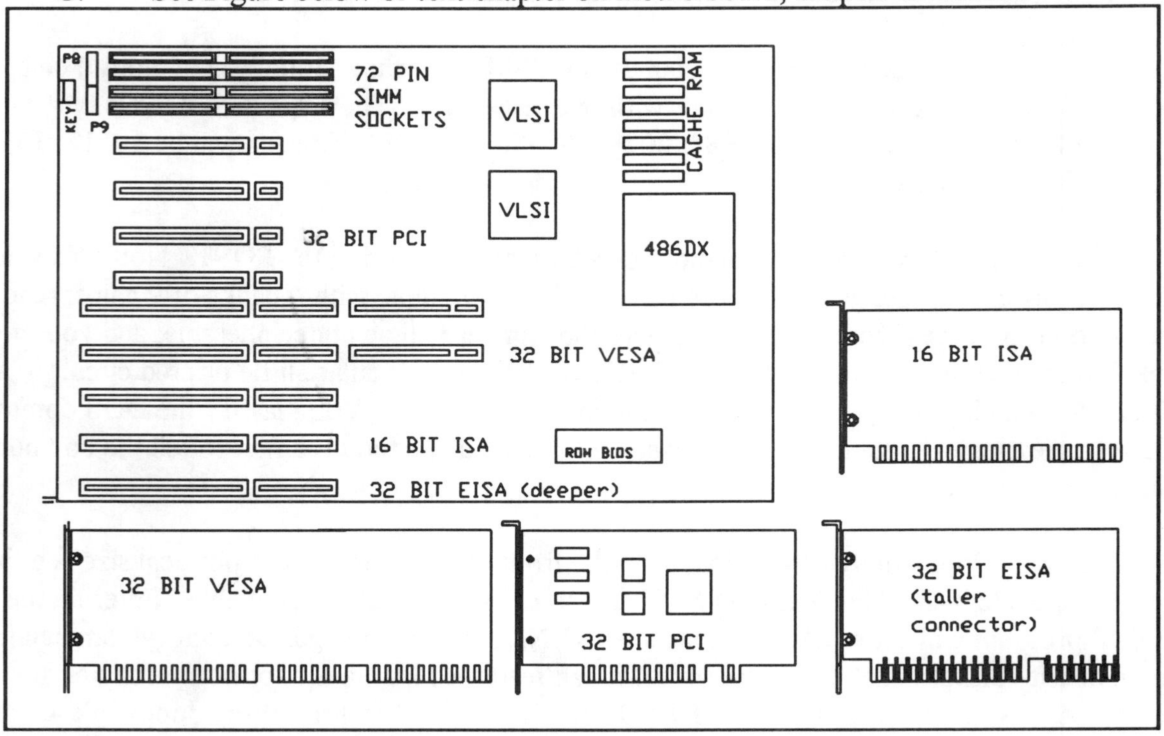

H. Look for dip memory chips separate from the RAM.

6. MicroSoft Diagnostics is a program included in DOS which gives system information. Type CD\DOS followed by an ENTER to change to the DOS directory. Then type MSD, and choose every option by typing the red or bold letter. Observe, but do NOT write down all information. Exit MSD by pressing function key F3. The following is the help screen from the MSD/? command

MSD [/B] [/I] [/F filename] [/P filename] [/S [filename]]

/B Runs MSD in black and white instead of color (for monitors that can't correctly display MSD in color).
/I Specifies that no initial hardware detection be performed(used if MSD does not start up correctly).
/F filename Writes complete MSD report to specified file.
/P filename Writes complete MSD report to specified file, without requesting any user input.
/S [filename] Writes summary MSD report to specified file. If no filename is specified, output will be to screen.

7. Run MicroSoft Diagnostics again using the following command. The F parameter or switch means put the information in a file on disk. SYSINFO is just a filename for the file holding

system information.

MSD /F sysinfo

8. Using the command "TYPE sysinfo | more" command, examine the system information MSD has given you.

9. Use the MEM command to glance at RAM memory usage. The following is the MEM/? help screen.

MEM [/CLASSIFY | /DEBUG | /FREE | /MODULE modulename] [/PAGE]

/CLASSIFY or /C Classifies programs by memory usage. Lists the size of programs, provides a summary of memory in use, and lists largest memory block available.
/DEBUG or /D Displays status of all modules in memory, internal drivers, and other information.
/FREE or /F Displays information about the amount of free memory left in both conventional and upper memory.
/MODULE or /M Displays a detailed listing of a module's memory use. This option must be followed by the name of a module, optionally separated from /M by a colon.
/PAGE or /P Pauses after each screenful of information.

10. Use the SCANDISK program to examine the file structure of the main hard drive. Do NOT do a surface scan. CHKDSK is quicker and more concise.

11. Examine the AUTOEXEC.BAT file with the "TYPE C:\autoexec.bat | MORE" command.

12. Examine the CONFIG.SYS file with the "TYPE C:\config.sys | MORE" command.

REPORT FOR LABORATORY 1

Name: ________________________ Date: __________ Class: _____________

PURPOSE:

____

____

____

____

____

____

____

OBSERVATIONS:

____

____

____

____

____

____

____

____

PROBLEMS ENCOUNTERED:

____

____

____

2 USING METERS

PURPOSE: To give the student their initial exposure to analog and digital meters, and logic probes, and gain experience measuring voltage and resistance.

EQUIPMENT:

analog meter
digital meter (use both types if possible)
digital logic probe
variable lab power supply
various resistors, labeled or have color code chart
47 Ω, 1 KΩ, 2.2 KΩ, 47 KΩ, 330 KΩ

PROCEDURE:

1. Following instructors explanation of equipment, set power supply to varied outputs as given in table 2.1 using only the power supply meter or settings. If test leads are not already connected to your meter, insert the red lead in the meters positive voltage jack (usually indicated with a +), and the black lead in the meters negative jack (usually indicated with a - or "com" for common or ground). Using the your meter, you will measure this voltage, and note in table 2.1. With voltage, POLARITY is important, so always connect the positive lead to the positive terminal, and the negative lead to the negative terminal. Set meter FUNCTION switch to DC VOLTAGE, and RANGE switch to value ABOVE the voltage expected. To measure, connect the red test lead to the positive terminal of the power supply, and the black test lead to the negative terminal.

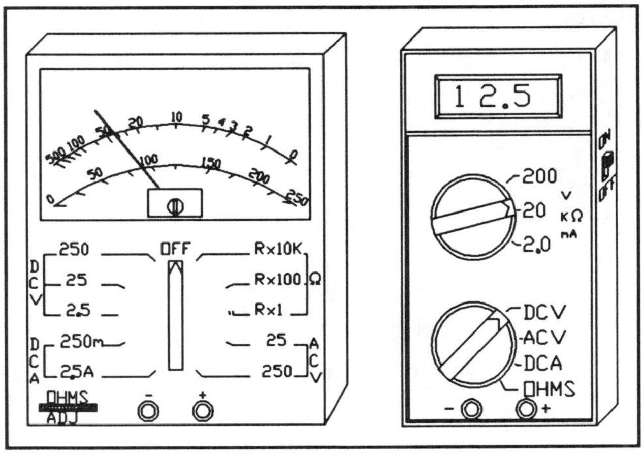

On the digital multimeter (DMM, right in figure), lower the range until 3 significant digits are displayed. If you go down one more range, the meter should show an OVERRANGE signal of some kind, often a 1 with no zeros to the left, but blanks. On the analog meter (left in figure), lower the range until the needle is in the middle 2/3 of a scale. Choose the correct scale, and read the value. If you have both kinds of meters, compare the readings. For measuring a negative voltage with the analog meter, reverse the leads, using red for the common or ground. The DMM automatically measures negative voltage, so you do not have to reverse the leads. Note your readings in table 2.1.

Table 2.1

VOLTAGE, POWER SUPPLY METER		VOLTAGE, DMM/ANALOG METER
1	.8 volts	
2	2.0 volts	
3	5.0 volts	
4	11.5 volts	
5	-12.0 volts	

2. Resistance is how difficult it is for electrical current to get through an object. On resistors, there is no polarity, so you can measure in either direction, and the red and black lead are interchangeable. The unit of resistance is OHMS. You will measure five resistors, and note the values in table 2.2. Set meter FUNCTION switch to RESISTANCE (the greek symbol Ω is often used for ohms). On the analog meter, in the OHMS position, the range scale is actually a multiplier, such as R*1 or R*10, meaning multiply the reading times 1 or 10. Set range to the highest setting. Place the test leads across a resistor. With the analog meter, bring the range down until the needle is in the middle 2/3 of a scale. Choose the correct scale, and read value. Multiply this value by the resistance multiplier on the range scale. This is the value of the resistor. On the digital meter, bring the range down until a 1 is alone on the left of the display. This is TOO LOW of a range. Go back one range for the most accurate reading. The reading is the resistance, there is no need to multiply.

Use a resistor color code chart or ask instructor the correct value of the resistor. Values over 1000 ohms are divided by 1000 and given the unit KILO-OHMS or Kohms. Match each resistor to a line in table 2.2, and measure and note. Compare your reading to the color code value.

Table 2.2

	OHMS , RESISTOR COLOR CODE	OHMS, DMM/ANALOG METER
1	47 ohms	
2	1000 ohms	
3	2200 ohms or 2.2 Kohms	
4	47 Kohms	
5	330 Kohms	

4. The logic probe is meant to measure just two voltage levels, high and low. A low is zero volts, and a high is 5.0 volts. In practice, these can range from 0.0 to 0.8 volts for a low, and 2.0 to 5.0 volts for a high. Somewhere in between .8 and 2.0, the low to high transition occurs. High and low are usually indicated by different colored LEDs (Light Emitting Diodes). Do **NOT** use the logic probe on voltages above 5 volts.

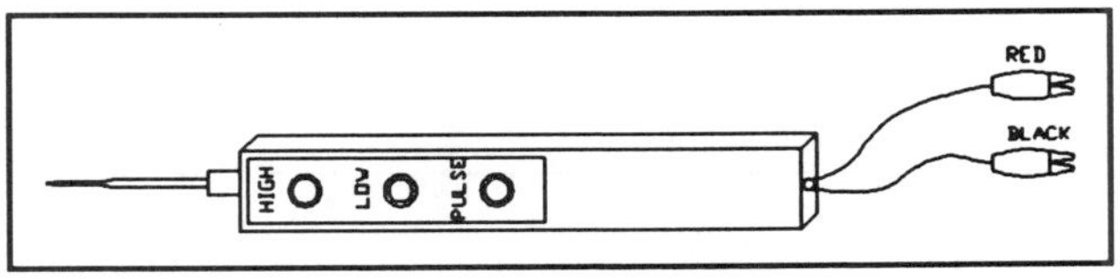

You can set one supply on the variable supply to 5.0 volts D.C. This is to power the logic probe. Connect the red lead of the probe to the positive (+) terminal of this supply, and the black lead to the negative (-) terminal. Now touch the probe tip to the positive supply and the HIGH LED should light. Touch the probe tip to the negative supply and the LOW LED should light. If you have a dual supply, touch the probe to the positive terminal of the second supply, and vary it from 0.0 to 5.0 volts, noting the response of the probe in table 2.3.

Table 2.3

	VOLTAGE RANGE	HIGH or LOW LED
1	0.0 to 0.8 volts	
2	0.8 to ?.? volts	
3	?.? to 2.0 volts	
4	2.0 to 5.0 volts	

REPORT FOR LABORATORY 2

Name: ____________________ Date: __________ Class: ____________

PURPOSE:

OBSERVATIONS:

PROBLEMS ENCOUNTERED:

3 SYSTEM ASSEMBLY & TEST LAB

PURPOSE: To give the student their first experience disassembling a total system, reassembling it. We use a working system to avoid some possible difficulties (interrupt conflicts), and assure controller and device compatibilities.

EQUIPMENT:

Functioning system
toolkit
bootable DOS disk with mem and chkdsk

REMEMBER:

1. Never install or remove anything with power on.
2. Wear the antistatic wristband when handling boards. Attach it to bare metal case.
3. Never FORCE a board or drive in any way.
4. Never touch the edge card connectors. Hold boards by edges or rear bracket.

PROCEDURE:

1. Make careful notes on the system set up shown in the ROM BIOS message on boot up, jumpers, and front panel switch connectors. Extremely carefully, note the AC power cord connections from the power supply to the front panel switch if one exists. Note the connections of the floppy drive controller cable and the hard drive controller cable(s). Remember pin 1 is usually identified by a red or blue stripe on the ribbon cable, or a triangle sign on the connector of the cable. On the cards, the end pins often have a silkscreened number 1,2 or 33,34. On the copper side (not component side), pin 1 often has a square pad instead of a round one. If the drive controller is a combined floppy/hard controller, note which cable is which.

2. Turn the system on to verify operation before you disassemble. Go into the system SETUP (often hold down DEL while booting) and note all settings. Of course, turn it OFF before continuing.

3. Totally disassemble system. No two parts should remain together. DO NOT REMOVE ANY CHIPS FROM THE BOARDS! Unplug all major subassemblies such as the keyboard, display, and mouse from the system. Make additions to your notes as you proceed, so you can reverse the procedure. Remove:

   a. case cover. (4 to 6 screws on rear of case)
   b. video card (one screw on top of rear bracket). Always touch a card only by the bracket or edges. Have anti-static wristband on or touch the bare metal of the supply to discharge static.
   c. serial-parallel-multi I/O card if present.

d. floppy and hard controller cards, disconnecting cables first, and noting pin 1 and cable placement.
e. any other cards, keeping careful notes on cable placement and pin 1.
f. power cables from all devices and motherboard. Note colors of wires going to Plug 8 and Plug 9 (front and rear) so you are positive which goes where. They are polarized so they only fit one way. Never force any plug.
g. the floppy drive(s), cables are already off controller card. Note which end the "twist" is on, and which plug (if two) goes to which drive.
h. the hard drive. Treat this VERY gently. Mechanical shock can destroy a hard drive. This is a good time to note the MAKE & MODEL.
i. the power supply. (4 or 6 screws on rear of case)
j. the front panel connectors to the motherboard. Note these carefully!
k. the mother board. (one screw in right rear of board, by keyboard jack and slide board and plastic standoffs to left and lift. They sit down in holes, and then slide right to install.)

4. Reassemble the system according to the steps learned in lecture. Do all intermediate tests. Compare all audio and video error codes (beeps) to the list in the book. Install:

a. motherboard sits down with plastic standoffs in holes of bottom of case, and slides right with plastic standoffs in slots. Usually there is only one screw into a metal standoff on the right rear. Connect the front panel cables from notes.
b. power supply (unless it is the way of the drives). Connect power supply cables to P8 and P9 from notes. An error on these cables could damage the motherboard. If the supply goes to a front panel on/off switch, be very careful to reconnect properly, as this is 110VAC, and dangerous.
c. connect power supply to wall, and turn system on. You should here beeps from the speaker. These are audio error codes, but are a GOOD sign here for they mean the motherboard is running well enough to complain that nothing is plugged in. Power down (turn off the system).
d. Insert the video display adapter card into an I/O connector usually farthest from the drives to keep it out of the way. Plug the display into the card and the wall.
e. power up the display, then the system. Beeps should be heard, and errors show on the display. What they say is not important yet. Power down both.

The purpose of powering up each time is to see if the last installed device is operational. If it is not, or the system is not, you know the device causing the problem. The alternative is to install everything, turn the system on, and if it is dead, or severely malfunctioning with no error codes, you have more trouble finding which device is causing the problem. As you gain more experience, you can build farther along before testing, perhaps after all basic devices are installed, and before any exotic ones are.

f. Insert the floppy drive controller card in a slot near the drives.

g. install the floppy drive(s), connect power supply plugs, and controller card cables, carefully using observation and notes for proper placement and pin 1 alignment.
h. install the hard drive controller near the drives.
i. install the hard drive, connect power supply plug, and controller cable from notes.
j. install multi I/O and other cards, and connect mouse.

5. Check all connections, and turn on the system. Note any audio or video error codes. If there are any, correct what you can, then consult instructor.

6. Use the c:\dos\chkdsk command to test the hard drive and the floppies.

7. Use the c:\dos\mem command to show memory usage.

TROUBLESHOOTING:
Audio and video error codes are given in Appendix A.
The following is the sequence of observable actions by the system.

a. hear or feel the fan begin
b. see keyboard LEDs flash from power up
c. hear the hard drive wind up and spin
d. see video card ROM message on screen
e. see system ROM BIOS header on screen
f. hear the POST RAM memory test and see it on the display (CMOS SETUP may allow turning audio clicks on or off, and testing memory above 1 meg)
g. see keyboard LEDs flash from POST
h. see drive A: LED and hear head seek
i. see drive B: LED and hear head seek
j. see hard drive C: LED
k. hear one beep of POST confirming all OK
l. see system ROM BIOS configuration message on display (usually showing installed equipment and memory)
m. booting from hard drive
n. see a starting MS-DOS message
o. see a few messages from the config.sys file
p. see a few messages from the autoexec.bat file
q. see a C:\> prompt if you have a hard drive or see an A:\> if you have a bootable floppy in drive A:

From the above, we can develop a troubleshooting strategy. Follow the following sequence of events carefully, noting the systems behavior. This should give clues to any problems. If there is an obvious error code or problem, jump in at the correct point below.

1. Power up the system. Is the display power indicating LED on? Is the fan of the power supply of the system spinning? Did the keyboard LEDs flash. If so power supply is probably OK. Is the hard drive winding up with an audible spin, and does it head seek after wind up? If so, the power supply is definately OK, and the hard drive physically OK. If not, use a meter and check the power supply (next lab), or replace the power supply.

2. Now the video card ROM message (if it gives one) should appear on the screen. Then the system ROM BIOS header stating what bios is running appears. If these do, the video is obviously at least basically functioning. If not, check the seating of the video controller card, that the type of card matches the display type, and the brightness and contrast settings of the display. [You have already checked that the display power LED is on, and the motherboard color/mono switch in the wrong position will not stop the display from working, and neither will the CMOS SETUP, which you can't see anyway if the display doesn't work.]

3. Now the POST does a RAM check and this is shown on the screen and clicks on the speaker. Your CMOS SETUP may allow turning audio clicks on or off, and testing memory above 1 megabyte of memory. This test confirms the RAM is installed and operating OK. If not, check the type and size of RAM chips, and their seating. Check documentation on chip placement.

4. The keyboard LEDs will flash a second time now, as the CPU senses if the keyboard is properly connected. This does not test each key, but is just an overall confirmation that the keyboard is OK. If they do not flash, you may still wait for an audio or video error code, as the system will either continue its initialization, or as for an F1 to continue.

5. The A: floppy drive is now turned on and a head seek done. If this occurs, the floppy is at least partially OK. If not, note this for future checking.

6. The hard drive LED should light, showing it is being accessed. Then ONE beep should sound showing the system is basically OK. This is the end of the POST. If a sequence of long and short beeps is heard, carefully note it, and look it up in the audio or video error code listing.

7. The ROM BIOS now should show a configuration message on the display showing the equipment installed and how much memory. Note the CMOS SETUP of all drives. If this does not appear, some error message should. If the CMOS SETUP has not been done, do it now. You usually enter it by pressing the DELete key at this time.

8. If DOS has been installed on the hard drive, it should start now, running the config.sys and then the autoexec.bat. If DOS has not been installed, then you should have a bootable floppy disk in drive A:, and the system will boot from that.

9. If the system gets this far, you can run a complete diagnostic program from floppy drive A: if desired. To test a drive's basic functions without a diagnostic program:

a. make the drive to be tested the default drive by typing "A:" and pressing ENTER for drive A:. The prompt should be A: now.
b. copy a text file from another drive by typing "COPY C:autoexec.bat" or any other filename you know exists.
c. now see if it was indeed copied and can by read by typing "TYPE autoexec.bat" or whatever file you used.
d. repeat for all drives. This is a reasonable basic function test.

All keys on the keyboard except the function keys and the screen movement keys can be tested reasonably well by just pressing all the keys one at a time at the DOS prompt. If they appear on the screen, they are working.

RAM can all be tested by using the advanced CMOS setup and choosing to test ram above 1 meg. If that option is not available, insert the line DEVICE=C:\DOS\HIMEM.SYS in your config.sys and boot again. Himem tests extended memory.

REPORT FOR LABORATORY 3

Name: ______________________ Date: _________ Class: ____________

PURPOSE:

OBSERVATIONS:

PROBLEMS ENCOUNTERED:

4 POWER SUPPLY LAB

PURPOSE: To learn to fully test the power supply.

EQUIPMENT:

multimeter
functioning computer system
toolkit
load resistor(s)

PROCEDURE:

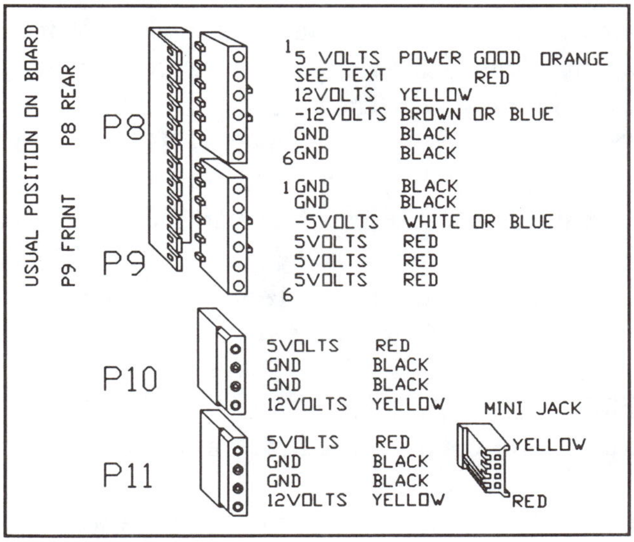

1. Boot your system, and note the power supply switch, fan operation, and sound at a distance. The muffin fan is usually powered by the +12 volt supply. If it is running, 90% of supply is OK. Is the supply "WHINING" ? This may show it is under too heavy of a load. A computer supply must be plugged into some device to work (motherboard, drive, dummy load). It can not be properly tested unloaded.

2. Turn OFF your system, and remove the cover. Trace the supply cables, noting what devices or peripherals it supplies. Reboot the system, and use a multimeter to test the voltages of plugs 8 and 9 against the proper values. If access to P8 & P9 (6 pin plugs) is difficult, hidden under the power supply or something, then just test one of plugs 10-13 (4 pin plugs for floppy, hard, or CD rom drives), on which red is +5v and yellow is +12v. The 5 volt supply should be above 4.75v and below 5.25 volts. The 12 volt supply should be above 11.5 volts, and below 12.5 volts. For positive voltages, touch the black or negative lead to one of the black ground wires in plug P8 or P9, and the red or positive lead to the pin to be measured. For negative voltages, Use the DMM the same way, but switch leads on an analog (needle) meter. Note voltages on the lines below.

JACK	REAR P8						P9						FRONT
PINS	1	2	3	4	5	6	1	2	3	4	5	6	PINS
	5	5	12	-12	GN	GN	GN	GN	-5	5	5	5	
	ora	red	yel brn	blu	blk	blk	blk	blk	wht	red	red	red	
MEASURED VOLTS	___	___	___	___	___	___	___	___	___	___	___	___	
WITH LOAD RESIS	___	___	___	___	___	___	___	___	___	___	___	___	

3. Turn OFF your system. Note on PAPER the wiring of an external, front mounted power switch. It is critical to replace these EXACTLY the same way. Now remove the power supply. In some cases the floppies in front of the supply must be removed first, to make room to slide the supply forward to disengage a bottom slot from the tab on the bottom of the case. Connect supply to the load resistor and measure the voltages again. Note these measurements in the second row above. The load resistor allows you to test power supplies without using a system. The load resistors can become very **HOT**. Examine the physical attributes, read the manufacturers label, reinsert the supply. When replacing supplies, these physical attributes (the form factor) must be carefully matched. Be careful the polarity of the plugs is correct. NEVER force the plugs on the mother board. (**Do NOT open the supply , it contains dangerous voltages. Only electronic technicians should open the supply.**) Have the instructor check the wiring of the 110vac power switch BEFORE you power the system back up.

TROUBLESHOOTING:
Audio error code = repeating short beeps, Video error code = 100

1. The motherboard, or an adapter card, or a drive could be pulling the power supply voltages down. The supply usually senses a low voltage, and shuts itself off. If the power supply is really "dead", there can be no other symptoms, as the system will be dead also. Check AC from the wall. If the display is plugged in there, and the display pilot LED is on, the wall plate has power. Check the fan. If it is running, the supply is 90% OK. If the fan is not running, you still do not know if the supply is "dead" or something is loading it down too much to run.

2. Measure the voltages at P8 & P9 with the motherboard attached. If the voltages are good, the power supply is OK. If not, then disconnect P8 & 9 and connect a load resistor pack, or a KNOWN good motherboard or drive for a load. Measure again. If the voltages are correct this time, something was pulling the power supply down. Reconnect the supply and remove one adaper card or drive at a time, powering up in between, until the fan comes on. The last item removed was the culprit.

3. If you have no meter, just replacing the supply with a KNOWN good one may be the fastest thing to do.

REPORT FOR LABORATORY 4

Name: ______________________ Date: _________ Class: ____________

PURPOSE:

OBSERVATIONS:

PROBLEMS ENCOUNTERED:

5 MOTHERBOARD LAB

PURPOSE: To be able to identify components and connectors of motherboard, remove it, and replace it.

EQUIPMENT:

functioning computer system
bootable DOS diskette
tool kit
bad motherboard from lab box labeled"bad motherboards"
soldering kit (if facilities permit)

PROCEDURE:

1. Cold boot the system to confirm operation. Note (ON PAPER) the CMOS setup for drives, if one exists. Turn system OFF!

2. Remove cover of system. Note CPU type and speed, and I/O slot type. Carefully document motherboard connections from:

a. power supply
b. case front panel connectors from
   1. speaker
   2. reset switch
   3. keylock switch
   4. turbo switch and L.E.D.
   5. power L.E.D.
   6. hard disk L.E.D. (to HDD controller card)
   7. system speed L.E.D. read out if any.
   8. any other connectors.
c. metal screws and plastic standoffs from case.

3. Protect the system from static discharge. Remove I/O adapter cards. Find and remove screw(s) holding motherboard to case bottom (usually one, sometimes two or more) and then the remove the motherboard by sliding the plastic standoffs from the slots and then lifting the board up and out. Examine it closely, identifying as much as possible, including:

ram
cache ram
rom BIOS
keyboard rom
cpu
npu math coprocessor socket

CMOS battery
crystals
type of I/O connector slots

4. Replace the motherboard, sliding it in with the plastic standoffs in position. Secure with the screw(s) into the metal standoff(s). Using original notes, reconnect all connections to the motherboard. Be very careful that the metal standoff touches only the proper area of the motherboard, and does not short it out. Power up the system to confirm operation. If the system does not come up, strip out all except for keyboard and video card, and use troubleshooting from total system assembly and test lab.

5. **Get a motherboard from the lab box labeled "bad motherboards.** Note position and orientation of each of the above chips. The NOTCH identifies pin 1. **Do not remove the chips from the good motherboard.** With permission of the instructor, using extreme care and an anti-static wrist band, remove each removable chip one at a time from a BAD motherboard, and replace before removing the next. Watch for leads bent under, or out.

6. Observe the instructors desoldering and resoldering demonstration. **Get a motherboard from the lab box labeled "bad motherboards.** Using the soldering kit, carefully remove the CMOS battery. Let the instructor examine the job. Then replace the battery, and again let the instructor examine the job.

TROUBLESHOOTING:
Audio error code = 1 long and 1 short beep, Video error code = 1xx

1. Check voltages to motherboard from power supply.

2. Confirm RAM installed properly.

3. Check voltage of CMOS battery.

4. You may swap out any socketed chip with a KNOWN good, identical motherboard.

5. If you ever throw away a motherboard, keep all socketed chips for future swapping. Watch for static electricity.

REPORT FOR LABORATORY 5

Name: ______________________ Date: __________ Class: _____________

PURPOSE:

OBSERVATIONS:

PROBLEMS ENCOUNTERED:

6 KEYBOARD LAB

PURPOSE: To learn to diagnose problems in, disassemble, and repair keyboards.

EQUIPMENT:

Functioning system
multimeter
non-working keyboard**(if available from lab "bad keyboard box")**
hobby knife
soldering kit (soldering iron, sponge, solder, solder wick)
wire
diagonal cutters
wire stripper
tool kit
(optional) oscilloscope, female 5 pin din jack, 5v power supply

REMEMBER:

1. XT/AT switch setting
2. CMOS setting (installed)
3. cable continuity

[A new keyboard is now about $20. Is it worth repairing?]

4. dust - 1 or 2 keys failing with NO pattern
5. PCB trace broken - 2 or 3 keys failing in a PATTERN
6. replace keyboard - electronic failure
7. replace Keyboard bios - if new keyboard does NOT fix problem.

PROCEDURE:

1. Confirm operation of keyboard by typing "DIR" for a directory.

2. Change CMOS setting to NOT INSTALLED. Reboot, test keyboard. Note symptoms of failure. Return CMOS setting to INSTALLED. Reboot.

3. Power down. Change keyboard XT/AT switch to WRONG setting. Power up. Note symptoms of failure and error messages. Power down and reset correctly.

4. Set multimeter to RESISTANCE function, and the lowest range. Disconnect it from the system. Remove the back of the keyboard.
Test continuity of cable.

5. If a working junk keyboard is available **(from the lab box labeled "bad keyboard box")**,

test to confirm operation. Open and identify a PCB trace that goes to 2 or 3 keys. With a sharp hobby knife, cut the stripe. Power up and Note PATTERN of keys failing. Power down and solder the stripe back (may need jumping with small wire). Power up and confirm operation.

6. Confirm overall operation of keyboard. Open system, determine if system has a separate, socketed keyboard BIOS rom. If so, remove, power up, and note symptoms of failure and error messages. Power down, replace, power up and confirm operation.

7. Plug the keyboard into the female 5 pin din jack, and connect the +5volts and ground to pins 5 and 4 as shown below.

TABLE 12.1 KEYBOARD SIGNALS ON MOTHERBOARD JACK
(shown in figure 12.1 with keyboard unplugged)

PIN	SIGNAL
1	5 volts Keyboard clock, pulled high
2	5 volts Keyboard data out pulled high
3	5 volts keyboard reset, pulled high
4	0 volts ground
5	5 volts power from motherboard

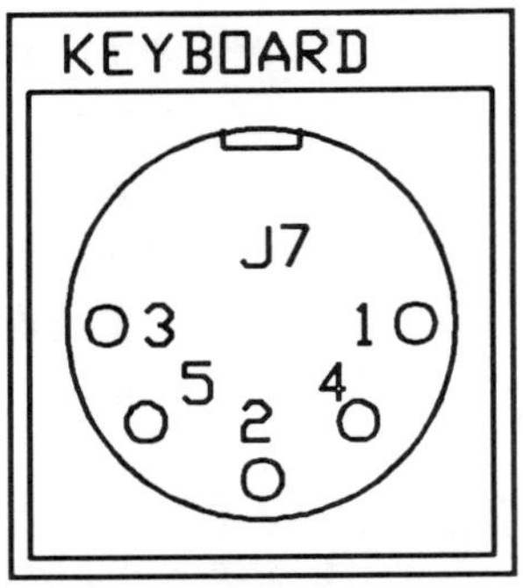

Figure 12.1 Keyboard Jack

Connect the oscilloscope ground to pin 4, and the probe to pin 2. Set the vertical sensitivity to 1 volt/division, and the horizontal time base to .1 millisecond/division. Set coupling at DC, and the Trigger to normal. Hold down a key for a stable repeating pattern. Note the difference between the key patterns. These are the actual bits of the key scan code. Compare to the code in the text. Note the keyboard is sending serial data, so this pattern is similar to the serial pattern shown in the section on serial ports.

TROUBLESHOOTING:
Audio error code = two short beeps, Video error code = 300

1. For $20, or even $16 for a NEW keyboard, you can't spend much time fixing an old one. Check the AT/XT switch if one exists on the bottom of the keyboard. Check the CMOS SETUP for the keyboard being installed.

2. If the keyboard appears dead, replace with a KNOWN good one.

3. If one or two random keys are not functioning, suspect dirt, and blow out with compressed air.

4. If a pattern of keys are failing, suspect a broken trace. If you are good with a meter and soldering, you may attempt a repair, using continuity checks. Keep the figure $16 in mind!

REPORT FOR LABORATORY 6

Name: ______________________ Date: _________ Class: ___________

PURPOSE:

OBSERVATIONS:

PROBLEMS ENCOUNTERED:

7 COMPUTER DISPLAY LAB

PURPOSE: To learn to identify, install, and test various displays.

EQUIPMENT:

Functioning system
bootable DOS disk
diagnostic program(s)
different types of displays with matching controller cards
tool kit

PROCEDURE:

1. Set up a functioning system with the DISPLAY MONITOR(s) to be examined.

2. Identify the monitor by noting:

a. physical size of screen ________________ inch diagonal

b. plug at the end of cable ________________ pin

c. front panel controls ________________

____

____

d. rear panel controls ________________

____

____

____

____

____

2. Attach display to system. Setup system for proper display (mono,CGA,VGA) with motherboard jumper (or switches) and in CMOS setup (if 286 or higher). Turn on system.

3. Listen for AUDIO ERROR CODE

1 long, 2 short
1 long, 3 short
1 short, 1 long with bad video
1 short with bad video)

a. Audio error code noted ________________

4. Note any VIDEO ERROR CODE (display is 4xx) see Appendix A.

a. Video error code noted ________________

5. Change Setup system for display (mono,CGA,VGA) with motherboard jumper (or switches) and in CMOS setup (if 286 or higher) to **WRONG** setting. Reboot and note audio and video error codes. Correct settings when done.

6. Run a diagnostic program to test the adapter and monitor.
(Checkit and QaPlus are two standard diagnostic programs.)

a. To run Checkit, type "CHECKIT". At the main menu, use the arrow key to move the menu to "TESTS" . Arrow down to "VIDEO" and run tests. When done, at main menu, arrow to "BENCHMARKS", arrow down to "VIDEO", and run. When done, arrow to "EXIT", and press RETURN to exit.

b. To run QaPlus, type "QAPLUS". At main menu, arrow to "TESTING". Under the testing menu, arrow down to "VIDEO", and run. When done, at main menu, arrow to "EXIT", and press RETURN to exit.

TROUBLESHOOTING:
Audio error code = 1 long 2 short beeps, Video error code = 400 mono, 500 color
1 long 3 short beeps
1 short 1 long & bad video
1 short & bad video

1. Unless you are a trained electronic technician, do not open a display. It has dangerous voltages. Stick to front and back panel adjustment controls. Is the display ON/OFF switch on? Is the pilot LED on? If so the wall has power, and the display power supply is working. Are the brightness and contrast controls all the way up (or at least in the middle of their range)? If you can feel static from the screen attract the hair on your arm when you rub your arm on the screen, or if the screen will hold a small piece of paper to it, the high voltage is working. If it will not do these however, it does not absolutely prove the high voltage is not working.

2. Is the motherboard video switch in the correct position, color/mono. Is the CMOS SETUP display set to the correct type? These will not stop the display from working, but just

give an error message.

3. Does the video adapter card match the display? Are there any rear bracket switches on the adapter card? If so set them according to documentation.

4. Is the video adapter ram in place and well seated.

5. If there is still no video, replace the video adapter card, and then the display itself. Fuses in the display monitor are often soldered in, and often require removal of a circuit board to reach. The CRT and capacitors can store enough charge to be dangerous. Do not open a display unless you are an experienced technician.

REPORT FOR LABORATORY 7

Name: ____________________ Date: __________ Class: ____________

PURPOSE:

OBSERVATIONS:

PROBLEMS ENCOUNTERED:

8 FLOPPY DRIVE LAB

PURPOSE: To learn to diagnose, remove, install, and test floppy drives.

EQUIPMENT:

Functioning system, bootable DOS disk
diagnostic program(s), toolkit
disk with bad FAT table (purposefully made)
scratch disk (formatted, data will be destroyed)

PROCEDURE:

HARDWARE FAMILIARIZATION

To gain experience with floppy drives, remove the cover of your system, and if necessary the drive(s) to get clear views of the heads and internal circuitry. Check off each of the following as you accomplish that task.

1. Identify the head positioning motor and mechanism. ____
2. Identify the spindle motor. ____
3. Identify the write protect sensor. ____
4. Identify the track zero sensor. ____
5. Identify the high density media sensor (if 3.5 HD) ____
6. Identify the index sensor. ____
7. Identify the Drive Select Jumper. ____
8. Identify the Diskette Change Jumper (if HD) ____
9. Identify the terminating resistor (if it exists) ____
10. Note twist in cable (count lines twisted) ____
11. Note cable END for A: (does it have termination R) ____
12. Note cable CENTRAL connector for B:(is it NOT term) ____

DRIVE INSTALLATION
(system with no floppy drives installed)

1. If there are jumpers on floppy controller card, set per documentation, then connect the cable noting pin one by colored wire on ribbon. Insert in I/O slot close to drive bays.
2. Set jumpers on floppy drive for second drive select, as in DS1.
3. Mount drive in case drive bays, A: is usually mounted in the top bay.
4. Connect power cable and data cable.
5. Check connections, power up system.
6. Enter the CMOS SETUP program and set floppy drive(s) to what you installed.
7. Reboot. Do a DIR on a floppy in the drive.

8. Do a CHKDSK A: on a floppy in the drive.
9. A real test of the drive is to read a professionally written diskette, as in a purchased program to check head alignment, and then to write a diskette and read it on another drive. This confirms compatibility of the drive with other systems.

SOFTWARE FAMILIARIZATION

With floppies functioning, run the diagnostic program(s) supplied, selecting full floppy drive tests on all floppy drives. Diagnostic programs may have to be loaded on and run from the hard drive to test the floppy drives.

To gain experience with DOS programs, you need a DOS diskette with command.com, msd, chkdsk, recover, scandisk, and attrib programs. You should also have a "BAD" diskette. A "SWITCH" is a parameter to follow the command.

1. Boot from floppy A: with DOS diskette. Do a DIRectory ____
2. Run MSD. This is not really a diagnostic, but gives information about the system. ____
3. Do a CHecKDiSK of this DOS diskette (no switches) ____
   Use SCANDISK for DOS 6.2 and above.
4. Look over the information this gives you. ____
5. Insert your "BAD" diskette in the other drive ____
6. Do a CHecKDisk on this diskette (no switches) ____
7. Look over the information this gives you. ____
8. Do a CHecKDisk on this diskette (with /F switch) ____
9. Look at the FILE0001.CHK that was created with TYPE ____
10. Do a CHecKDisk on this diskette (no switches) ____
    (This is to make sure it is FIXED)
11. With the COPY command, copy a file from drive A: to B:. Immediately open the B: drive DOOR (button/lever) while the pilot light is on (to RUIN the disk again). ____
12. Do a CHecKDisk on this diskette (no switches) ____
    (to confirm you have RUINED the disk again) ____
13. Do a RECOVER filename on the file you copied badly ____
14. Look at the FILE0001.REC with the TYPE command ____
15. Use the FORMAT B: command to make B: a DATA disk ____
16. Insert B: floppy in A: drive and try to BOOT ____
17. Insert the DOS disk in A: and BOOT ____
18. Use the FORMAT B:/S command to make a BOOTABLE disk ____
19. Use the DIR B: command to see what was transferred ____
20. Use the DIR B: /A:H to see the HIDDEN files transferred ____
21. Use the command /? switch with FORMAT, CHKDSK, RECOVER, TYPE, and DIR to see short HELP file. ____

TROUBLESHOOTING:
Video error code = 600

1. Confirm proper seating of controller card. Confirm cable has 7 twisted wires, and drive A: is at the end of the cable, B: second from the end. Jumpers set on drive for DS1 out of DS0,DS1, or DS2 out of DS1,DS2. Check for termination resistors if needed, and connections to power supply. Check CMOS SETUP of floppy drives.

2. Try a "DIR" command with a KNOWN good floppy of the proper density in the drive. Watch for the drive access LED to light and the spindle to spin.

3. If it is a used drive, you may clean heads and try again.

4. Swap floppy controller, cable, and drive one at a time with KNOWN good ones.

5. If this fails, strip the system to bare bones, nothing but keyboard, video card & display, floppy controller and drive, and power supply connected to motherboard. Have all the front panel display lines disconnected. Try the above again.

REPORT FOR LABORATORY 8

Name: ______________________ Date: _________ Class: ____________

PURPOSE:

OBSERVATIONS:

PROBLEMS ENCOUNTERED:

9 HARD DRIVE LAB

PURPOSE:

To learn to diagnose, remove, install, and test hard drives.
To be able to identify 506, IDE, and SCSI drives by sight.

EQUIPMENT:

Functioning system with hard drive.
Bootable diagnostic diskette (qaplus and checkit)
toolkit
2 scratch disks
bootable DOS diskette(s) with at least the following programs:
attrib, backup, chkdsk, command.com, defrag
debug, fdisk, format, mem, msd, recover,
restore (or MSbackup), scandisk

PROCEDURE:
(system without hard drive installed yet)

1. Identify your drive. We low level format ONLY MFM/RLL drives.

   ST506 MFM/RLL ____
   IDE ____
   SCSI ____

2. Identify your drive parameters, Capacity, Cylinders, Heads, Precomp, and Sectors.

3. Set any jumpers on the hard drive controller card per documentation. Connect cables noting pin 1. Insert in open I/O slot close to drive bays. Mount the drive in a bay (often a hidden bay with no opening to the front of the case) and connect power, data, and control cables.

4. Check connections, power up the system, enter the CMOS SETUP and set the drive parameters according to your documentation. Reboot with a bootable DOS diskette in floppy drive A: with at least fdisk, format, and debug.

WARNING: STEP 5 & 6 ARE FOR ST-506(mfm,rll) TYPE DRIVES ONLY!! Check with your instructor!

5. Using DEBUG, attempt to access the HARD DRIVE CONTROLLER BOARD ROM to low level format the drive [if MFM or RLL].

   DEBUG
   g=C800:5 or CC00:5 or CA00:5 or C800:CCC

6. Whether or not that is successful, now use CHECKIT to low level format the drive [if MFM or RLL].

7. Now use FDISK to partition the drive [this is destructive of information already on the drive]. Use the FDISK command to "display" information about the partitions. Note if they are "active" (can be booted).

8. Use the DOS FORMAT/S command to high level format the drive. [this destroys old data]. Use the ATTRIB command to display file information including hidden or system files.

9. Use CHKDSK to see information on hard drive.

10. Use BACKUP or MSbackup command to save hard drive data to floppies.
    BACKUP C:\ A:/S
    or
    BACKUP C:\subdirname a:
    Msbackup is controlled with the TAB, SPACEBAR, and ENTER keys.
    If you select more than 1.4 Megs of files, you will need more than 1 floppy.

11. Use the RESTORE command to transfer that backed up info back to the hard drive.
    RESTORE A: C:\/S
    or
    RESTORE A: C:\subdirname

12. Copy 10 or so small (10-20K) files to a floppy. Now erase 2 or 3 at various positions in the directory listing, but not the first or last. Now run Defrag A: and see the gaps in the sectors. Exit Defrag. Now copy a 100k or so file to A: and run Defrag A: again. Note that the large file was split into pieces to fit into the small gaps. Now run the Optimize selection and watch how the disk is "defragmented". This is done on a floppy because a hard drive could take an hour or more.

13. On the floppy, run Scandisk, and note the operation. It may be run on the hard drive also, but the "surface scan" could take an hour or more.

TROUBLESHOOTING:
Video error code = 1700

1. Confirm jumper settings, cables polarity by pin 1, proper cables.

2. Check card pressed down in I/O slot,

3. Boot system, watching for audio and video error codes. It they appear, look up meaning and attempt to correct. Listen for spin up and head seek, which at least confirms the drive is physically capable of functioning. Go into CMOS SETUP to verify proper parameters against documentation.

4. Boot from floppy, run FDISK to access drive. If it will not, run a diagnostic program to attempt a low level format. This destroys old data, and is not advisable on an IDE drive, unless your program is designed for that specific drive.

REPORT FOR LABORATORY 9

Name: ________________________ Date: __________ Class: ____________

PURPOSE:

OBSERVATIONS:

PROBLEMS ENCOUNTERED:

10 GAME PORT (JOYSTICK) INSTALLATION

PURPOSE: To gain experience installing game ports and interfacing joysticks.

EQUIPMENT:

Game port adapter card, or Multi I/O card with Game Port
Game port test software, or Game
Joystick
functioning system
toolkit

PROCEDURE:

1. With the power off, remove the case cover from the system. Use an anti-static wriststrap, or touch the bare metal of the power supply to discharge static electricity from your body before proceeding.

2. Select an open I/O connector (expansion slot), and remove the rear metal bracket covering the slot opening in the case. Insert the card carefully but firmly. Secure it with a screw in the top.

3. Connect the joystick to the Female DB15 connector on the rear bracket. Replace the case cover. Power up.

4. Install the game, or testing software you have available according to instructions that come with the software. Run the game. This may entail changing to the game subdirectory with a CD\GOLF command (for a game called golf), and doing a DIR *.EXE and DIR *.BAT for an executable file or batch file to start the game. For example, GOLF.EXE or GOLF.BAT.

TROUBLESHOOTING:
Video error code = 1300

1. Check proper seating of adapter card, and connection of joystick.
   Check for MIDI port on sound card that may conflict with joystick.
   You may have to disable one or the other.

2. Check for proper installation of software that uses joystick.

3. Run MSD to see if it detects a game adapter under "OTHER ADAPTERS"

4. If it does not, try a different game adapter card.

REPORT FOR LABORATORY 10

Name: ________________________ Date: _________ Class: ____________

PURPOSE:

OBSERVATIONS:

PROBLEMS ENCOUNTERED:

11 SERIAL PORT INSTALLATION LAB

PURPOSE: To successfully install an RS-232 series communication port.

EQUIPMENT:

- A functioning system
- a serial adapter card
- diagnostic programs
- toolkit
- serial loopback connector

PROCEDURE:

1. Run diagnostic to examine interrupts and DMAs and I/O addresses already in use. Choose an available IRQ.

2. Open case of system. Inspect for existing serial ports.

3. Using anti-static procedures, install the new adapter card in open slot. Use 8 bit slot if possible, to save 16 bit slots for future use by 16 bit cards. The usual IRQs follow.

SERIAL RS232 PORTS ADDRESSES AND INTERRUPTS

PORT	I/O ADDRESS	INTERRUPT
COM1:	3F8H TO 3FFH	IRQ4
COM2:	2F8H TO 2FFH	IRQ3
COM3:	3EBH TO 3EFH	IRQ4
COM4:	2E8H TO 2EFH	IRQ3

Note that IRQs can be possibly be shared, but only by devices that are not in use at the same time. Test both devices thoroughly to confirm operation. The serial port can be tested with a LOOPBACK plug which tricks the computer into thinking a device is connected. A simple COPY CON: COM1: command followed by a line or two of text, and a control Z, will complete a test.

4. Using a loopback connector, test the port. Pinouts follow in case you need to construct the connector.

SERIAL LOOPBACK PLUG 25 PIN AND 9 PIN

STANDARD 25 ALTERNATE 25 9 PIN

line	2 - 3	line 2 - 3	1 - 4 - 6
	4 - 5	4 - 5	2 - 3
	4 - 6	6 - 8 - 20	7 - 8
	20 - 8		
	20 - 22		

Note, when the computer sends a Request To Send on 4, it gives itself a Clear To Send and a Data Set Ready on 5 and 6. When the computer sends out a Data Terminal Ready on 20, it sends itself a Carrier Detect and Ring Indicator on 8 and 22. The Data it sends on 2, it also receives on 3.

5. You must set up the com ports with the following DOS command.

MODE COM1:BAUD,PAR,DATA,STOP parity = Even, Odd, None. Data bits = 7 or 8. Stop = 1 or 2. As an example:
MODE com1:1200,n,8,1

6. The port may be tested with a diagnostic program, or a simple DOS test. COPY CON: COM1:. After this type two lines of text. Then enter CONTROL Z, as you learned to do with the copy command. If it says ONE FILE COPIED then it successfully wrote out the port.

TROUBLESHOOTING:
Video error code = 1100

1. Check serial adapter card jumper settings and seating.
   Check any internal devices that may conflict, such as scanner, serial mouse, fax/modem.

2. Run MSD to see if it detects the card port.

3. Use the loopback connector for tests with diagnostic software.

REPORT FOR LABORATORY 11

Name: ______________________ Date: _________ Class: ___________

PURPOSE:

OBSERVATIONS:

PROBLEMS ENCOUNTERED:

12 MOUSE LAB

PURPOSE: To properly install mouse in system.

EQUIPMENT:

mouse
mouse adapter card (or existing, unused serial port)
mouse software
functioning AT system
Dos
diagnostic software

PROCEDURE:

1. Read mouse installation instructions that come with the mouse.

2. Note existing serial ports on system for possible interrupt conflicts.

3. Cold boot system and confirm operation with DIRectory on hard and floppy drive. **Turn OFF system.**

4. Confirm interrupt setting, and insert mouse adapter card in open slot. (For serial mouse, connect to serial port).

5. Create mouse subdirectory (CD\mouse), and copy mouse software from floppy to hard drive in mouse subdirectory.

6. Insert **c:\mouse\mouse.com** command in autoexec.bat or **c:\mouse\mouse.sys** command in config.sys. (See EDIT below)

7. Warm boot the system to activate the autoexec.bat and config.sys files.

8. Enter the **EDIT** program to test mouse by moving mouse and observing corresponding movement of cursor.

9. Run a diagnostic program to confirm interrupt usage.

10. Remove commands from autoexec and config files. Power down system.

11. With power **OFF**, remove mouse adapter card and mouse from system.

SERIAL MOUSE INSTALLATION.

1. Identify COM1: and COM2: on your system. Determine which, if either, is being used. Watch for modems, which use a COM port. If your motherboard does not have serial ports on board, you may need to install a dual serial adapter card. Many systems have a MULTI I/O card with two parallel, two serial, and a game port. Find out what you have and write it down for future documentation.

2. Plug your mouse into the serial port chosen. If your system has 25 pin D shell connectors, you may buy adapters to change the output from 25 to 9 pin.

BUS MOUSE INSTALLATION

1. Set the interrupt setting on the BUS board to an UNUSED interrupt irq 2-5. Interrupts for 8088 systems are found in table 3.6. Interrupts for 286 and above systems are found in table 3.8. On a PC/XT 8088 system board, 5,6,7 are hard drive, floppy drive, and lpt1: parallel printer port respectively. That leaves 2, 3,and 4. IRQ4 is for com1: so if you have a serial port, that is gone. IRQ3 is for com2: which may be open, and IRQ2 is perhaps your most likely choice. On an AT (286 or above), IRQ14 is used for the hard drive, and IRQ5 is used for a second parallel port lpt2:. If you don't have a second parallel port, then IRQ5 is open. So IRQ2, 5, or 3 are the most likely choices.

2. Install the Bus board in an expansion slot and plug in mouse. Avoid using expansion slot 8 on an XT.

SOFTWARE INSTALLATION FOR BUS AND SERIAL MICE

Most peripherals are well documented, and come with software that automatically installs itself. Just read the manual, follow the installation instructions, and everything will go nice and easy. Just in case that doesn't work, I offer the following.

Since mice are the first peripheral we are covering that needs its own software to drive them, I give two lists below showing you how to install the drivers. You should refer back to these lists for most of the following devices also. The first list is for automatic installation. This may or may not be included with your software. The second list is for manual installation.

AUTOMATIC DEVICE DRIVER INSTALLATION.

1. Change the active drive to A:

    A:

2. Find the name of the program.

    DIR *.EXE

DIR *.COM
DIR *.SYS
One of these should give a program with a recognizable name, like install.exe or setup.exe.

3. Run that automatic installation program.
INSTALL (or SETUP)

MANUAL DEVICE DRIVER INSTALLATION.

1. Create a subdirectory with an appropriate name.
C:
MD\mousedrv

2. Change to that subdirectory
CD\mousedrv

3. Copy all the files from the floppy to the hard drive.
COPY A:*.* C: /V

4. Identify the driver.
DIR *.EXE (mouse.com or mouse.sys or similar)
DIR *.COM
DIR *.SYS

5. Mouse.com is run in the autoexec.bat file.
Mouse.sys is loaded in the config.sys file.
Edit each file as required. If you have no instructions from the documentation, for the serial mouse try a line similar to: MOUSE N where N is 1 or 2 for COM1: or COM2:

TROUBLESHOOTING:

1. Check for IRQ jumper settings and seating of card.
Check for conflicting IRQs on other cards.

2. Check for the software driver in the config.sys or autoexec.bat file.

3. Checkit does not have a mouse test, QAPLUS and AMIDIAGS have good tests for the mouse.

Usually the mouse package has detailed documentation and other programs for calibrating and testing the mouse.

REPORT FOR LABORATORY 12

Name: ______________________ Date: __________ Class: ______________

PURPOSE:

OBSERVATIONS:

PROBLEMS ENCOUNTERED:

13 DOT MATRIX PRINTER LAB 1

Using the Dot Matrix Parallel Printer

PURPOSE:

The purpose of this lab is to examine the different ways to output information to the parallel printer, and test its functionality.

EQUIPMENT:

a computer system, toolkit, a parallel loopback connector, a printer cable paper, diagnostic software, and a printer with documentation.

PROCEDURE:

1. Connect the printer to the parallel port of the system

2. Use the PRINT command to print out the autoexec.bat and the config.sys

3. Use the COPY CON: LPT1: command to print directly from the keyboard to the printer.

4. Use the SHIFT PRINTSCREEN command to print the screen to the printer.

5. Use the CONTROL PRINTSCREEN command to "toggle" printing on. Do a few DIRs. Use it a second time to "toggle" the printer off.

6. Use the HELP PRINT command, and the PRINT menu selection to print out the help file.

7. Use Qbasic to write a graphics program. or copy the following.

CD\DOS
Qbasic

Press ESCape key to get past information screen, then type the following lines.

```
screen 12           : rem this sets the display for graphics
circle (50,50),30,2 : rem this draws a circle.
```

Hold down ALT press R to get the RUN menu, then let go of ALT and press S for start. Note the screen should show a circle.

[For fancier effect, the program below may be used instead.]

```
SCREEN 12     : rem this sets the display for graphics
FOR R = 10 to 100 STEP 10 :rem this loops 10 times to next R
```

```
CIRCLE (320,240),2*r,r/10
REM the above draws circles of different sizes and colors
NEXT R.
```

8. Do a SHIFT PRINTSCREEN, AND note no circle is printed.
   Press any key to return to the program.
9. Press ALT F A for Save As and give a filename "circle".

10. Press ALT F X to exit.

11. Use the GRAPHICS command to set the printer up for graphics. You may have to do CD\DOS to get to the correct directory first.

12. Load and run the Qbasic program again, and do the printscreen again.

Qbasic
   Press ESCape key to get past information screen
      ALT F O   for open
      Tab to the filename circle.bas
      Press the space bar to select it
      press RETURN
      ALT R , S to run,

13. Do a shift printscreen now. Note the printer should print the circle.
   Exit Qbasic by pressing the ALT F, X, N keys.

14. Run MSD and note information on the parallel port.

15. With nothing at all connected to the parallel port, use the COPY CON: LPT1: command to try to send data out the parallel port. Note the error message. Now, using the parallel loopback connector, try sending the information again. No error message should be displayed.

16. With and without the loopback connector, run your diagnostic program, noting the results.

TROUBLESHOOTING:
Video error code = 900

1. Run MSD to detect and report on the parallel port.
   Check for conflicting devices with a diagnostic program.

2. Use a parallel loopback connector and run a diagnostic program.

3. Run the printer self test, often by holding down the form feed while turning power on. This will confirm the printer is functioning but not the printer interface to the computer.

REPORT FOR LABORATORY 13

Name: ______________________ Date: __________ Class: ____________

PURPOSE:

OBSERVATIONS:

PROBLEMS ENCOUNTERED:

14 DOT MATRIX PRINTER LAB 2

Repairing the Dot Matrix Parallel Printer

PURPOSE:

The purpose of this lab is to become familiar with the repair procedures for the common failure modes of the dot matrix printer.

EQUIPMENT:

Dot matrix printer with documentation, toolkit, paper.

PROCEDURE:

1. Run the printer self test. For many printers, this is done by holding the Form Feed button down and turning the printer power on.

2. Remove the paper.

3. Remove the ribbon.

4. Remove the print head.

5. Remove the upper case.

6. Remove the platen (rubber rolling pin). Stick on mailing labels often peel off the backing and get stuck in the printer paper path, causing paper jams. Check paper path for stick on labels.

7. Identify the paper out sensor. It should be a small switch, either mechanical of optical located in the paper path.

8. On the motherboard, identify:
    a. the low voltage power supply
    b. the microprocessor
    c. the ROM
    d. the setup switches
    e. the output transistor or chip (head driver)

9. Identify the:
    a. PLATEN drive motor
    b. HEAD drive motor
    c. friction/tractor drive selector switch
    d. darkness/multiple copy lever/switch

10. Remove the motherboard for replacement.

11. Reassemble the printer. Self test to insure operation.

REPORT FOR LABORATORY 14

Name: ______________________ Date: _________ Class: ____________

PURPOSE:

OBSERVATIONS:

PROBLEMS ENCOUNTERED:

15 LASER PRINTER LAB

PURPOSE: The purpose of this lab is to become familiar with a laser printer.

EQUIPMENT: Tool Kit, Laser printer

PROCEDURE:

Since printers differ, use documentation or ask the instructor to find the side the control panel is on, and the self test technique. The following uses an old HP compatible laser. For toner and cleaning, read your printers documentation carefully.

1. Do SELF TEST. [Power up Push round button on rear of left side.

2. Do TEST. [On control panel, Press On line to get OFF LINE, press TEST.

3. Open unit top half. [Lift up green lever on right side]

4. Remove & replace fixing (fusing) assembly cleaner. [With top up, flip fusing cover up and back, and slide cleaner out to right, Fig 3-12., replace.]

5. Remove toner cartridge. [With top up, flip down toner door on right side, slide toner cartridge out to right. Fig 3-10 Treat it gently! Do not invert! Do not expose light sensitive drum to light!, replace.]

6. Clean Primary Corona Wire. [With top up, toner cartridge out, remove green plastic square with felt brush. Carefully slide back and forth on top of cartridge. Fig 5-7. Reinstall brush and cartridge.]

7. Clean Transfer Corona Wire. [With top up, middle of bottom with zig-zag wires. Use cotton swab VERY CAREFULLY!! Fig 5-8.

8. Clean Transfer Guide. [Behind transfer corona wire. Use cloth! Fig 5.9]

9. Remove, Clean, Replace Paper separation belt. [VERY CAREFULLY!!! Watch orientation. Fig 5-10.]

10. Remove 4 screws of back panel. Remove back cover panel.

11. Remove 4 screws of top cover panel and three cables.

Remove top cover panel.

12. Remove 2 screws of left cover panel. Remove left cover panel.

13. Open right toner door, remove 4 screws and right cover panel.

14. Remove 2 screws on EACH SIDE of front cover and front cover.

15. Remove 1 screw and carefully fold up gray AC POWER cover.

16. On left rear PCB, Remove 4 top screws and one screw on outside left cover, and one screw with ground lug holding bracket on right side of PCB. Remove 3 cables and PCB.

17. Visually identify parts of the laser printer, including paper path. Fold down LOWER rear cover to expose rear of paper path.

18. Reassemble laser printer. Test!!

REPORT FOR LABORATORY 15

Name: ______________________ Date: _________ Class: ___________

PURPOSE:

OBSERVATIONS:

PROBLEMS ENCOUNTERED:

16 SOUND CARD INSTALLATION

with Windows Sound Recorder and Windows Media Player

PURPOSE: To gain experience in installing sound cards

EQUIPMENT: sound card, driver software, speakers, microphone
system with Windows, diskette with .wav files
sound card test program

PROCEDURE:

INSTALLING A SOUND CARD

1. Note the default settings on the berg shunt jumpers on your card. They are set at the factory to the most common settings.

2. Using MSD or a similar diagnostic program, identify the interrupts already used (see section 9.12 of text). Confirm Base I/O address and range, interrupt, and DMA the board is set for are available, or reset jumpers.

3. With system plugged into the wall, have power OFF. Remove the cover. Touch the exposed, non-painted metal of the power supply, or wear an anti-static wrist band.

4. Remove the metal back bracket by an empty I/O slot of the proper size (8 or 16 bit). After checking DMA, IRQ, and I/O ADDRESS settings, install card in the I/O slot. Plug in mike and speakers. Plug speakers into power if required. Power up system.

5. Install the driver software according to the manual for your specific sound card. Usually, just put it in A: drive, type A: enter, and INSTALL.

6. Run the test program, check volume control on card rear bracket. If OK, continue. If not, check settings, consult instructor.

7. In Windows, under Control Panel, choose Drivers. Under setup, you may set I/O address.

USING THE WINDOWS SOUND RECORDER

1. Type WIN to get into Windows

2. Under ACCESSORIES double click on Sound Recorder. The following symbols stand for the actions shown, much like an audio cassette recorder.

rewind	fast for	Play	Stop	Record
◂◂	▸▸	▸	◘	Mike

3. In Sound Recorder, click on the microphone symbol, and speak into the mike. Make sure the switch mounted on the mike is ON. Click on the square STOP button to stop recording.

4. Click on Stop, Rewind, and Play. Your recording should play back.

5. Click on File, Save As, and type in NAME.wav to save file to disk.

6. Insert lab diskette with .WAV files into drive A:. Click on File, Open, the diskette to change to A: drive, and one of the files shown ending in .WAV, and OK.

7. Click on Play ▸.

8. Click on Effects and experiment with each option.

9. Click on Edit and try each option. On Mix, remember to REWIND, then play.

10. Click on File, Exit when done.

USING THE WINDOWS MEDIA PLAYER

1. Type WIN to enter Windows

2. Under ACCESSORIES double click on Media Player. The following symbols stand for the actions shown, much like an audio cassette recorder.

Play	Stop	Rewind All	Rewind Step	Forward Step	Forward All	Fine Tuning
▸	■	|◂	◂◂	▸▸	▸|	◂▸
Pause						

3. Click on File, Open, Drive A:, a filename.WAV, OK

4. Click on Play button and you should here the sound.

5. Experiment with all other buttons.

TROUBLESHOOTING:

1. Check the IRQ, DMA channel, and Base I/O address jumpers or settings on the card itself. Check the speakers, microphone, and all else is connected to the proper jack on the card.

2. If other cards interfere, remove them and run MSD or a diagnostic program to detect actual IRQ, DMA, and I/O address of sound card. Then add the cards one at a time, running the diagnostic program each time to discover the IRQ, DMA, and I/O address of each card. Game adapters for joysticks may conflict with a MIDI port on the sound card. You must resolve any

conflicts.

3. Check config.sys and autoexec.bat for lines pertaining to the sound card. Using documentation that came with the card, determine if the driver settings match the hardware settings.

4. Among MSD, AMIDIAG, CHECKIT, and QAPLUS, only QAPLUS detects the presence of the sound card, reporting it's I/O address. The more popular cards have a test program included in their associated software.

5. For one of the more popular cards, the following two lines should be in the autoexec.bat file. A is for I/O address, I for IRQ, and D for DMA. SBPRO is the directory of the programs.

```
SET BLASTER=A220 I10 D1 T4
SET SOUND=D:\SBPRO
```

REPORT FOR LABORATORY 16

Name: ____________________ Date: __________ Class: ____________

PURPOSE:

OBSERVATIONS:

PROBLEMS ENCOUNTERED:

17 CD-ROM DRIVE INSTALLATION

PURPOSE: To gain experience installing CD-ROM drives

EQUIPMENT:

IDE CD-ROM drive with controller (sound) card & cables
functioning system

PROCEDURE:

1. Boot the system to note operation, and copy or print autoexec.bat and config.sys files. Copy each to a .BAK file to save the old files. Run a diagnostic program and examine the IRQs, DMAs, and I/O addresses in use.

1. With the system off, remove the cover and touch the power supply bare metal, or use a anti-static wrist strap. Install the sound card in an empty slot. Observing polarity (pin 1), connect the IDE controller cable to the controller card. If the card has more than one IDE connector, they may be labeled by the brand name of the drives they handle. Try to match the connector to your drive. The four (4) pin DC power plug needs to be plugged in to the CD-ROM drive for the +5 and +12 volts. The 40 pin IDE connector should have one end labeled with pin 1 or 2, and the other end with 39 or 40. The 40 conductor ribbon cable should have a red or blue stripe on the side for pin one. A four (4) pin audio connector needs to be connected from the drive to the audio card. There may be a single thick wire to connect the metal case of the drive to the computer case for grounding. As typical with IDE, a drive select or identity (ID) jumper which must match the ID on the IDE controller on the sound card. Connect the audio cable to the controller card.

2. Install the CD-ROM drive in an empty bay. Connect the power supply cable, the IDE controller cable, and the audio cable.

3. Boot the system. Run your diagnostic program again and examine the IRQs, DMAs, and I/O addresses in use. This should tell you the information for the card you have installed. Place the floppy with the driver software in drive A: and type A: ENTER to make A: the default drive. Type INSTALL or SETUP and press the ENTER key. Follow the prompts. You must REBOOT the system to put changes in the autoexec.bat and config.sys into effect.

4. Examine the autoexec.bat and config.sys files and note the changes or added lines the driver installation performed. If you have trouble and run the install program again, you should rem out the old lines in the config.sys and autoexec.bat files, to keep from having duplicate or similar lines.

5. Insert a CD into the drive, and use the DIR command on the drive letter you set the CD-

ROM drive to. You should see a normal directory.

6. If software was installed to test the drive, run it.

7. If the drive is not responding, check that the software installed the MSCDEX command in your autoexec.bat file. HELP MSCDEX will get you into the DOS help file on this command. Do read this if trying to install a CD-ROM drive. A typical line is as follows:

C:\DOS\MSCDEX.EXE /D:driver /L:E

where driver is the name of the driver program in your config.sys file, and E: is the letter designation of the CD-ROM drive.

8. Also check your config.sys file for a line accessing the driver that came with the drive. A typical line is as follows:

DEVICE=C:\DEVICEDRIVERS\ROMDRIVER.SYS /D:driver

where driver is the name given in the MSCDEX command in the autoexec.bat file.
The system must be rebooted, and the drive should now be able to be accessed just like another hard drive.

9. The documentation that came with your drive should have a troubleshooting section to refer to.

TROUBLESHOOTING:

1. Confirm IRQ, DMA, and I/O address of adapter card and all other cards. Check seating and polarity of cables to CD-ROM drive. Run a diagnostic program to confirm hardware settings. A Game adapter may conflict with the MIDI port on the sound card that also has an IDE CD-ROM controller.

2. Examine config.sys and autoexec.bat for lines pertaining to CD-ROM drive and note these. Compare to documentation that comes with the drive to insure these software settings match the hardware settings.

3. Run any test programs that came with the drive, and read the TROUBLESHOOTING or IN CASE OF TROUBLE sections of the documentation.

REPORT FOR LABORATORY 17

Name: ______________________ Date: __________ Class: _____________

PURPOSE:

OBSERVATIONS:

PROBLEMS ENCOUNTERED:

18 FAX/MODEM INSTALLATION

PURPOSE: To gain experience installing Modems / Faxes

EQUIPMENT:

Functioning system
Fax/modem kit with software

PROCEDURE:

1. Run a diagnostic program and examine the IRQs, DMAs, and I/O addresses in use. Check the documentation of your card to check the hardware settings on the card. Dip switches or shunt jumpers may set the COM port to be used. This must later be matched my the software settings.

2. Power down. Install the card in an empty I/O slot. Connect the phone jack in the wall to one connector on the rear bracket, and the phone to the other. The phone is not needed for the modem operation, and just daisy chained if needed to be used as a standard phone.

3. Power up. Run your diagnostic program again and examine the IRQs, DMAs, and I/O addresses in use. This should tell you the information for the card you have installed.

4. Place the software that came with the modem in drive A: and type A: ENTER, to make A: the default drive. If the software is self-installing, just type install or setup at the prompt. It will copy what is needed to the hard drive, and prompt you for settings. Often the software has a test mode or program.

5. Using the software documentation, enter a phone number of a local "bulletin board" to call. When the call is made, the speaker on the modem should allow you to hear the ringing, answering, and tones used. If you hear a person, then the modem on the other end was not in answer mode. If you hear "whistling tones" and then the speaker cuts out, you have connected. Most bulletin boards have a clear menu to follow, and you can quit when needed.

TROUBLESHOOTING:
Video error code = 6xx
1. Confirm the number you are calling, and that it has a functioning fax/modem in answer mode.

2. Run MSD or another diagnostic program to determine COM port and address used. Check card hardware jumper settings. Also check the usage of all other COM ports with a diagnostic program, to check for conflicts.

3. Check software settings of fax/modem program being run to confirm matching settings

with hardware.

4. Run any diagnostic program that came with the fax/modem, and refer to the troubleshooting section of the documentation.

REPORT FOR LABORATORY 18

Name: ____________________ Date: __________ Class: ____________

PURPOSE:

OBSERVATIONS:

PROBLEMS ENCOUNTERED:

19 OPTICAL SCANNER INSTALLATION

PURPOSE: To become familiar installing optical scanners.

EQUIPMENT:

optical scanner controller card
optical scanner
driver software
functioning system
toolkit

PROCEDURE:

1. Run a diagnostic program and examine the IRQs, DMAs, and I/O addresses in use. Check the documentation of your card to check the hardware settings on the card. Dip switches or shunt jumpers may need to be used to avoid interrupt collisions with other cards. This must later be matched my the software settings. Copy your autoexec.bat and config.sys files to .OLD or .BAQ files, to save. This allows you to check changes made by the installation of new driving software.

2. Power down and remove the case cover. Select an open I/O connector (expansion slot), and remove the rear metal bracket covering the slot opening in the case. Static electricity can damage the card or the motherboard, so use an anti-static writs strap, or touch the bare metal of the power supply to discharge your body. Insert the card carefully but firmly. Secure it with a screw in the top.

3. Plug the scanner into the jack on the rear bracket of the adapter card. Secure with a top screw, and replace the case cover. Power up.

4. Run your diagnostic program again and examine the IRQs, DMAs, and I/O addresses in use. This should tell you the information for the card you have installed.

5. Insert the driving software that came with the scanner in drive A: , and type A: ENTER to make A: the default drive. Follow the documentation on installing the software, or type INSTALL or SETUP. Most software is now self installing. Self installed software may be compressed or zipped, and require decompression or unzipping.

6. If your software is not self-installing, make a directory for it according to the suggestion in the documentation, or one that makes sense, like "SCANNER", with the command, MD\SCANNER. Change to this directory with the command CD\SCANNER. Now enter the command COPY A:*.* C:\SCANNER/V to copy all the files over to the hard disk.

7. Do a DIR RE*.* to find any "read.me" files that give information. Do a TYPE

READ.ME | C:\DOS\MORE command to print the file on the screen. You can also do this with any .DOC documentation file. Do a DIR *.EXE and DIR *.BAT to find programs that can be run. Run by typing the name.

TROUBLESHOOTING:

1. Check seating of card, and connection of scanner to card.
   Confirm IRQ, DMA, and I/O address of card with diagnostic program.
   Determine all IRQs, DMAs, and I/O addresses of other devices, to check for conflicts. Resolve any conflict by changing setting of one that conflicts.

2. Confirm lines in config.sys and autoexec.bat relating to the scanner match these values.

3. Verify you are using the correct settings and physical scanning technique with the scanner from the documentation that came with it. Most manuals have a troubleshooting section in case of problems.

REPORT FOR LABORATORY 19

Name: ______________________ Date: __________ Class: ____________

PURPOSE:

OBSERVATIONS:

PROBLEMS ENCOUNTERED:

20 TAPE DRIVE INSTALLATION

PURPOSE: To become familiar with the installation of the magnetic tape drive used for backup purposes.

EQUIPMENT: system, mag tape drive, driving software, formatted mag tape

PROCEDURE:

1. Because of the time required (1 - 2 hours) to format a mag tape, it is essential to have the tapes formatted before class. Copy your autoexec.bat and config.sys files to .OLD or .BAQ files, to save. This allows you to check changes made by the installation of new driving software. Have documentation for your particular drive close at hand.

2. Set jumpers or switches according to documentation. Physically mount the drive in an open bay, removing any front plastic bezel. Connect the power and signal cables, paying attention to pin 1.

3. Install software:
   a. boot the system.
   b. place the floppy containing the drivers in a drive.
   c. use the DOS command A: or B: to make that the default drive.
   d. type "install" or do a DIR *.EXE to find the name of the installation program.

4. Configure software for specific system hardware. This may be semi-automatic. Usually this will just be answering a list of questions the software asks you.

5. The tapes need to be formatted by the system. This can take two hours. Be sure these have been preformatted for you.

6. Select only a few files to be backed up. These may be copies you have made for safety. Run the backup software.

7. Erase the files you backed up.

8. Restore the files from the backup tape.

9. Return the system to its original state.

TROUBLESHOOTING:

1. Check cable connections and power to drive if external, and connection to floppy cable if internal.

2. Examine autoexec.bat and config.sys to see changes made by software.

3. Most software will give error codes or messages. Look these up in the documentation that came with your specific drive.

REPORT FOR LABORATORY 20

Name: ________________________ Date: __________ Class: _____________

PURPOSE:

OBSERVATIONS:

PROBLEMS ENCOUNTERED:

21 DOS LAB

PURPOSE: Initial familiarization with DOS. If familiar with DOS, skip this lab. It is located here because a basic familiarity with DOS is needed to proceed with future labs.

EQUIPMENT: functioning system, DOS installed

PROCEDURE:

1. Boot the system. It should arrive at a "C>" or "C:\>" prompt. This means DOS is running. Any internal or resident command will be run right from the DOS command interpreter named "command.com" which is loaded in memory. Any external or transient command is a separate program under the DOS directory.

2. Type "DIR" and press the RETURN or ENTER key. Note the names of files fly by on the screen. Try two ways to get help. Type "DIR /?". A screen of syntax should appear. This is a quick, sparse help screen.

3. Now type "HELP DIR". The HELP command gives much more information than the question mark switch. You go into an editor and can use the PageUp or PageDown keys or up and down arrow keys to move up and down through many pages of information. If there are angle brackets <> around any phrase, you may arrow to the first letter and press return (enter) to go to that related topic. There are three main sections of the help file on a command. You enter the "SYNTAX" section. The TAB key will move you from "NOTES" to "EXAMPLES", to the "<bracketed>" subtopics. Press ENTER at any of these to go to that section of help. The ESCAPE key backs you up to the section you just came from. Together these sections contain many pages of help on the command you asked for. You may print the help out to your printer with ALT F for FILE, and pressing "P" for print. Function key F3, or ALT F, X will get you out when you want to quit.

4. Typing "HELP" alone at the DOS prompt gives you an index, or list of all the topics available. Browsing this can be quite interesting.

5. The minimum commands you should try are:
ATTRIB, CD, CHKDSK, CLS, COPY, DATE, DEL and ERASE (on a junk file created with the COPY command), DIR, FIND, FORMAT (on scratch floppies, do NOT format C:), HELP, MD, MEM, MORE, MSD, PATH, PRINT, PROMPT, REN, RD (on a junk directory you created with the MD command), SCANDISK (do NOT do a surface scan), SORT, TIME, TREE, TYPE, VER, VERIFY, VOL, and XCOPY.

6. The EDIT command runs a word processing program. It is complex, so instructions are given here. It can be used to create files you will need to configure systems. For now, use it to create a junk file, or a report on this lab.

USING THE EDIT PROGRAM TO CREATE FILES

With DOS version 5.0 or newer, the EDIT program is a screen oriented editor, and is a great improvement. If you have it, try it. Just type EDIT to start it. The following is a brief overview of commands to get you started. With the F1 HELP key, you can soon become proficient.

The MAIN MENU is listed along the top of the screen. The ALT key activates the MENU so that touching one of the letters highlighted gives a pop up menu. Now you either press one of the new highlighted letters, or ARROW down to a selection and press ENTER to choose it. The main menu with all the pop up menus popped up follows.

Files	**E**dit	**S**earch	**O**ptions
New	cu**T**	**F**ind	**D**isplay
Open	**C**opy	**R**epeat	help **P**ath
Save	**P**aste	**C**hange	
save **A**s	cl**E**ar		
Print			
e**X**it			

Note only one of these is actually visible at one time. There is an instruction line at the bottom of the screen you should pay attention to. Some keystroke commands follow.

HOME	moves cursor to beginning of line
END	moves cursor to end of line
INSERT	toggles between "typeover" or "insert" modes
DELETE	deletes character or selected text
TAB	moves forward through the "help" fields
SHIFT TAB	moves backward through the "help" fields
ARROW	moves one character forward or backward or one line up or down
SHIFT ARROW	blocks or selects characters for editing
CONTROL ARROW	moves one "word" forward or backward
ESCAPE	cancels or backs you down the command structure

Gain experience with all commands as time allows.

REPORT FOR LABORATORY 21

Name: ______________________ Date: _________ Class: ____________

PURPOSE:

____

____

____

____

____

____

____

OBSERVATIONS:

____

____

____

____

____

____

____

____

PROBLEMS ENCOUNTERED:

____

____

____

22 SYSTEM CONFIGURATION LAB

PURPOSE:

a 286 or higher functioning system with at least 2 Meg of RAM.
DOS on hard drive or floppy

EQUIPMENT:

a bootable DOS diskette with the following files:
himem.sys, smartdrv.sys, ramdrive.sys,
fastopen.exe, memmaker, mem
a diagnostic program (optional)

PROCEDURE:

1. Cold boot your system from the hard drive. On the hard drive, look for the above files with the dir command ,as in DIR HIMEM.SYS command. If they exist in the root, note that. If not, change directory to the DOS subdirectory with a CD\DOS command, and look for the files again.

2. If they are not on the hard drive, Create a DOS directory (IF ONE DOES NOT EXIST) with the MD\DOS command, change to it with the CD\DOS command, and copy them from the diskette (which you place in drive A:) with the following command at the C: prompt.

COPY A:\DOS\FILENAME

Do this for each file. When finished copying, REMOVE the floppy!

3. On the hard drive C: , rename your config.sys file (if it exists) to config.bak with the following command.

RENAME config.sys config.bak

This saves your existing file, but keeps it from running, allowing us to create our own and note it's behavior. When the lab is over, you may delete your new files, and rename the original file so the system is as you found it. At the end of the lab, use the command:

RENAME config.bak config.sys

4. Now warm boot your system (ALT, CNTL, DEL) and carefully note the information on the screen This should be with NO config or autoexec file.

5. Now using the COPY CON: FILE command, create a config.sys file with HIMEM with the following lines:

```
COPY CON: CONFIG.SYS
DEVICE = C:\DOS\HIMEM.SYS
^Z
```

If you did this correctly, the system will respond with "1 file copied", and a DIR C*.SYS command will show the file, and a TYPE CONFIG.SYS command will show it to contain the line starting with DEVICE. The HIMEM program manages the systems extended memory and High Memory Area (HMA), allowing you to use memory above 640K for SOME programs.

6. Warm boot from the hard drive and note the information shown. It should say "XMS specification, installed A20 handler number 1". If not, identify your error, or consult your instructor. Use the MEM command to see how memory was affected.

7. Now, using the COPY CON: command as in step 6, create a new config.sys file with an additional line.

```
COPY CON: CONFIG.SYS
DEVICE = C:\DOS\HIMEM.SYS
DOS=HIGH
^Z
```

This new line DOS=HIGH loads DOS in the HMA, saving conventional memory (0-640K). Check the config file as in step 6, and WARM BOOT again, NOTING the system response. Use the MEM command again, and note results.

8. In the manner of step 6, create the new config.sys file below.

```
COPY CON: CONFIG.SYS
DEVICE = C:\DOS\HIMEM.SYS
DOS=HIGH
DEVICE=C:\DOS\SMARTDRV.SYS 128
^Z
```

The new line creates a disk CACHE to speed up system performance. Size can be from 128K to 8192K (8 Megs). Here, we use 128K. Again, reboot and note system response. Use MEM command again and note response.

9. In the manner of step 6, create the new config.sys file below.

```
COPY CON: CONFIG.SYS
DEVICE = C:\DOS\HIMEM.SYS
DOS=HIGH
DEVICE=C:\DOS\SMARTDRV.SYS 128
```

```
DEVICE=C:\DOS\RAMDRIVE.SYS  128/E
^Z
```

The new command creates a ram or electronic disk drive named D: of 128 Kbytes. Size may be from 16K to 4096K (4 MEGS). The /e places it in extEnded memory. A /a would place it in expAnded memory. Again, reboot, note response, use MEM, note response.

10. In the manner of step 6, create the new config.sys file below.

```
COPY CON: CONFIG.SYS
DEVICE = C:\DOS\HIMEM.SYS
DOS=HIGH
DEVICE=C:\DOS\SMARTDRV.SYS  128
DEVICE=C:\DOS\RAMDRIVE.SYS  128/E
INSTALL=C:\DOS\FASTOPEN.EXE C:=40
^Z
```

The new line creates a cache to hold 40 file names and locations. It remembers files you open often, and can reopen them quickly, speeding system performance. Reboot, note response, use MEM, note response.

11. When the lab is over, rename the old config.bak file to config.sys as shown in step 3, and boot the system to prove all is back the way it was.

REPORT FOR LABORATORY 22

Name: ______________________ Date: __________ Class: ____________

PURPOSE:

OBSERVATIONS:

PROBLEMS ENCOUNTERED:

23 AUTOEXEC.BAT LAB

PURPOSE: To learn to create and run batch programs using DOS only.
To create a basic autoexecutable batch file.

EQUIPMENT:
system with DOS

PROCEDURE:

1. Using the cd\dos command, move to the DOS subdirectory. IF you are NOT familiar with the following commands, use them with the /? switch to see a help page, then try them.

cls, date, dir, mem, more, time, type, ver, vol

Now create a file named JUNK1 using the COPY CON: command, holding names. For example:

```
COPY CON: JUNK1
smith, dave 444-6666
jones, joe  222-4444
adams, sue  111-5555
zebra, mary 777-3333
^Z
```

(that's a CONTROL Z)
(note the numbers start in column 13)

Also create a file named CR with the following commands.

```
COPY CON: CR

^Z
```

In the second line you type only a RETURN or ENTER.

2. Using the COPY CON: FILENAME.bat command, create a batch file of a few lines using the commands above. Use only one command per line. For example:

```
COPY CON: DO.BAT
cls
date
time
dir/o/w
type junk1
ver
vol
^Z
```

Note the output on the screen. Note the commands are shown, then performed.

3. The SORT dos command alphabetically sorts a file line by line. /r means in reverse order, /+13 means sort by the character in column 13. The FIND command searches for a "string" in a file, line by line. /v means all lines EXCEPT the ones with the string, /n means to NUMBER the lines, /c means just give the COUNT of the lines found, /i means IGNORE the case. Use the /? switch to learn about the two DOS commands. Now use many versions of the commands, noting the output. (Use the < redirection symbol for input.) For example:

```
sort < junk1
sort/+8 < junk1
sort/+13 < junk1
```

Note this only prints to the screen, JUNK1 is NOT CHANGED. If you want to change JUNK1, use the > output redirection symbol also. For example:

```
sort < junk1 > junk1
```

The TYPE JUNK1 command will now show the file is CHANGED.

```
find "joe" < junk1
find/v "mary" < junk1
find/n "5555" < junk1
```

4. The PAUSE batch command prints "Strike a key when ready" and stops for you to read what is on the screen. Create a batch file or fileS using the pause batch command, and the two DOS commands, sort and find. For example:

```
sort < junk1 > junk2
type junk2
pause
sort/r < junk2 >>junk2
type junk2
pause                    (Note junk2 is erased and rewritten)
sort <junk2 >> junk2
type junk2
pause                    (Note junk2 is APPENDED)
```

Perhaps another file:

```
find /n "smith" < junk1
find "dave" < junk1
```

When you run these files, note how the pause command works.

5. The ECHO OFF batch command "hides" or stops the commands from being shown, cleaning up the output. The @ figure "hides" the echo off command which cannot hide itself. CLS clears the screen, giving a clean field for your file. The | pipe symbol pipes the output of one command into another. Create a batch file using these commands, with others you have learned. For example, the following may be named dt.bat for date and time.

```
@echo off
cls
date < cr > dt
time < cr >> dt
type dt | find "Current"
```

Line 3 uses the CR file you created above to give a RETURN or ENTER required after the command. It also creates the file DT which is a data file for the DT.BAT file. Line 4 APPENDS the time to that file. Line 5 types out only the lines wanted.

6. The DIR command has a /p switch to paginate. How can you view other TEXT or ASCII files one screen at a time? The MORE command does this. To create a file too large to fit in 24 lines, use the copy command as follows.

```
COPY junk1 + junk2 + junk1 + junk2  junk3
```

Be careful not to copy a file to itself or the error "Content of destination lost" will occur. The PROMPT command is powerful. The simplest use is to change the prompt line. Precede each of the following characters with a $ for the response shown. $ = $, T = time, d = date, p = path, v = dos version, g = >, l = < b = |, _ = CR/LF (new line), s = leading space, h = backspace, e = escape.

Now create a batch file to use the MORE command as follows.

```
@echo off
cls
prompt $d$s$t$ssYour Command Master ?
TYPE junk3 | more
```

7. The prompt command can be more powerful. Like date and time on screen when in DOS? Create a batch file with the following prompt command.

```
PROMPT $e[s$e[1;1H$e[K$e[1;28H$d$e[1;45H$t$e[1;50H$e[K$e[u$p$g
```

$e[s	saves the present cursor position
$e[1;1H	moves the cursor to 1,1
$e[K	erases from cursor to end of line
$e[1;28H	moves cursor to 1,28
$d	writes the date
$e[1;45	moves the cursor to 1,45
$t	writes the time
$e[1;50H	moves cursor to 1,50
$e[K	erases cursor to end (seconds erased in this case)

$e[u	returns cursor to saved position
$p	gives path
$g	gives greater than sign

You see the prompt command can be very powerful. It can also control the color of the text and background.

8. One typical use of batch files is the AUTOEXEC.BAT which DOS runs automatically when booted. In it you can include the batch file above, and build your own menus. Create the following batch files.

```
rem     name this one wp.bat
@echo off
cls
echo    This is my word processor
pause
men
^Z

rem     name this one ss.bat
@echo off
cls
echo            This is my spread sheet
pause
men
^Z


rem name this one men.bat
@echo off
cls
echo
echo
echo                    Word Processing
echo
echo                    Spread Sheet
echo
prompt $
^Z
```

Now if you type men, it should put your menu on the screen. Typing WP or SS (the CAPS) [You could have numbered them 1, 2, and NAMED them 1.bat and 2.bat] should (fake) run your program. For really running programs, replace all the "ECHO" line in WP.bat and SS.bat with lines to change to the proper subdirectory, run the program, and change back to the root directory. For example:

cd\wp51	(for Word Perfect 5.1 directory)
wp	(to run it)
cd\	(to change back to root directory)

8. The AUTOEXEC.BAT file is run by the system each time you boot the computer. Some commands typically used in the autoexec.bat file are:
cls, date, doskey, echo off, path, prompt, time, and verify on.
Use each of these and any others your instructor suggests in a batch file. Run it by typing the name.

9. On the hard drive C: , rename your autoexec.bat file (if it exists) to autoexec.bak with the following command.

    RENAME autoexec.bat autoexec.bak

This saves your existing file, but keeps it from running, allowing us to create our own and note it's behavior. When the lab is over, you may delete your new files, and rename the original file so the system is as you found it. At the end of the lab, use the commands:

    RENAME autoexec.bak autoexec.bat

10. Create an autoexec.bat file or rename the one you created in step 8. Boot the system to see your file in action.

11. As mentioned in step 9, rename the original autoexec.bat file so the system is as you found it. Boot to make sure this is true.

CONCLUSION:

Batch files can be very powerful. We have just scratched the surface here. Autoexec.bat can bring your computer up on booting to some automatic process. With other batch files, it can MENU drive your system. It can automatically load and run BASIC programs on booting. The DOS batch commands make a programming language all its own!

REPORT FOR LABORATORY 23

Name: ______________________ Date: _________ Class: ____________

PURPOSE:

OBSERVATIONS:

PROBLEMS ENCOUNTERED:

24 DIAGNOSTICS LAB

PURPOSE: To become familiar with at least one professional diagnostic program.

EQUIPMENT:

diagnostic programs (QAPLUS functions shown below)
post diagnostic add in card with documentation

PROCEDURE:

1. Examine the following pages for the pull down menu structure of QAPLUS. Some of the functions are NOT available on this 360K disk. With QA diskette in drive A:, type A: if needed to get to the A: drive. Type QAPLUS to run the diagnostic program.

2. Under HELP, just observe selections. These are not available because of space.

3. Under REPORTS, just observe selections.

4. Under SYSINFO, do all except LOG.

5. Under INTERACT, do bad chip location, keyboard test, speaker test.

6. Under TESTING, do RUN TESTS.

7. Under SETUP, you may change things, but change them back so the system is functional when you are done.

8. Under UTILITY, QAclean is a head cleaning program, but it needs a special diskette. DO NOT do ANY of these!!!

USING THE POST ADD IN DIAGNOSTIC CARD

1. Carefully read the instructions that come with your card.
Turn system OFF !!!

2. Carefully insert your card in the correct orientation.
WARNING !!! INSERTING IT BACKWARD CAN DESTROY THE CARD!

3. Remove floppy and hard drive controller cards to create a problem.

4. Attempt to boot system and note operation of POST card.

5. Create other problems (correctable) and see what the card reports.

REPORT FOR LABORATORY 24

Name: ______________________ Date: _________ Class: ___________

PURPOSE:

OBSERVATIONS:

PROBLEMS ENCOUNTERED:

25 WINDOWS INSTALLATION

PURPOSE: To gain experience in installing Windows

EQUIPMENT: Windows installation diskettes

PROCEDURE:

Windows version 3.1 and 3.11 comes on six 1.44 Meg floppies which are numbered and have instructions on the label. The process is automatic and simple.

1. Insert disk #1 in drive A:

2. Type A: and press ENTER to make A the default drive.

3. Type "SETUP" and press ENTER to start the automatic installation process.

4. When done, type "WIN" to start Windows.

5. Exit Windows by holding down the ALT key and pressing F, then letting go of the ALT key and pressing X, then pressing the ENTER key.

6. If you are unfamiliar with Windows, the next lab will get you started.

REPORT FOR LABORATORY 25

Name: ______________________ Date: __________ Class: ____________

PURPOSE:

OBSERVATIONS:

PROBLEMS ENCOUNTERED:

26 WINDOWS LAB

PURPOSE: Initial familiarization with Windows

EQUIPMENT:

functioning system 386 or up with 2 or more Mbs
Windows installed, with mouse

PROCEDURE:

The Windows program has it's own tutorial included. You will run the tutorial to become familiar with Windows.

1. Boot the system. At the DOS prompt type "WIN". This will cause Windows to run.

2. The PROGRAM MANAGER should be on the screen. A header or title bar should be close to the top, with the following words.

FILE OPTIONS WINDOW HELP

Use the mouse to move the pointer to "FILE" and click the mouse button once. A small "pull down" menu should appear. Use the mouse to move down to "RUN" and click once. A window should appear.

3. Type WINTUTOR and press the ENTER key. This should run the windows tutorial. From then on just follow instructions.

[Instead of steps 2 and 3, you may just hold down the ALT key and press F for file, then R for run, and WINTUTOR and press the ENTER key.]

IF WINTUTOR WAS SUFFICIENT, YOU MAY STOP HERE.

4. MINIMIZING, MAXIMIZING, MOVING, and RESTORING WINDOWS

A window has a BORDER on each side and top and bottom, a negative sign in the top left corner called a CONTROL-MENU BOX, little up and down arrows in the top right corner called SIZING BUTTONS. The up arrow MAXIMIXES the window, or makes it take up the whole screen, and the down arrow MINIMIZES the window, or shrinks it temporarily out of the way. Clicking the mouse once on this minimized icon will bring up a menu. The Restore option makes the window go back to the size it was before it was minimized. The top right corner of a maximized window has a little double arrow, pointing up and down in the same square. The little down arrow is the RESTORE arrow, to go back to the size it was before maximizing. The Move option lets you relocate the window by dragging it where you want it. The Maximize option makes it fill the screen. The Close option makes it go back down to an icon. The Next option selects the next program. Instead of clicking once on an icon, and getting a menu, you may double click (click twice fast), and the window will open to the size it was before minimizing.

5. USING MENUS

Somewhere in the opening window, four icons should appear labeled Main, Accessories, Games, and Startup. Double click on the Main icon. In the Main window, double click on file manager with an icon of a two drawer file cabinet. A window should appear with a row of pull down menu subjects at the top. File, Disk, Tree, View, Options, Window, Help. To select a menu, hold down the ALT key and press the underlined letter you choose, or just click once on your choice. A menu should appear beneath the subject. To leave that menu without doing anything, either select another, or press ESCape. To select from the menu that appeared, click on your selection or press the underlined letter, no ALT key needed this time. To leave FILE MANAGER at this time, Press ESCAPE until you are at the beginning file manager window, and then press ALT F for file, and X for exit, or click on FILE and then EXIT. Or click on the control-menu box (the negative sign in the top left corner), and click on Close. This should bring you back to the original screen you had when Windows started.

6. SIZING WINDOWS

Double click on any icon to open a window. When it comes up in a window, move the cursor with the mouse to the bottom right corner, getting the cursor arrow point exactly on the border corner, so the cursor changes from an arrow to a two headed arrow at a 45 degreee angle. Now click and HOLD the left mouse button. This is like grabbing the corner of the window. Holding the left button down, move the mouse, and watch the size of the window change, being trimmed or expanded from the bottom right corner. This press, move, and let go is called dragging. The top and bottom and both side borders work exactly the same way to allow you to change the window to any size you like.

7. RUNNING MULTIPLE PROGRAMS

Double click on File Manager. Size this window to about 2x3 inches. Now click and HOLD on the title bar in the top row, between the minus sign on the left, and the down arrow on the right. Move the mouse, and you will see that you can move the whole window to any location you like. Let go of the button to leave the window where you want it. Now to open a second program at the same time, double click on README.WRI. This is a small information file for you to read. For now we are just using it as another window. Grab the bottom right corner and make it smaller. grab the title bar, and move this widow so both it and File Manager are visible, though they may overlap. Now double click on Control Panel. When it appears, make it smaller, and move it where you want it. Now click anywhere in any of these windows, and note the title plate become blue or dark. This means this window is active now. You can click in any window, and work in it, then click in another and work in it.

8. EXITING WINDOWS

To exit Windows, close any open windows first by clicking on the control menu box (the little negative sign in the top left corner of that window, and clicking on close. When all are closed, do the same to the Program Manager. Windows gives you a last chance to change your mind, then exits.

REPORT FOR LABORATORY 26

Name: ______________________ Date: __________ Class: ____________

PURPOSE:

OBSERVATIONS:

PROBLEMS ENCOUNTERED:

APPENDIX A - POST ERROR CODES

POST AUDIO ERROR CODES

These beeps from the system speaker are given by many BIOS during POST (Power On Self Test).

AUDIBLE BEEPS FROM SPEAKER (Audio Error Codes)	POSSIBLE ERROR
1 short beep, system works	All OK
no beep, dead unit continuous beep repeating short beep	Power Supply
1 short, continuous	First bank of RAM
1 long, 1 short	System motherboard
1 long, 2 short	Display
1 long, 3 short	Display
1 short, 1 long, bad video	Display
1 short, bad video	Display
1 short, video good, no boot	disk drive

POST VIDEO ERROR CODES

These numeric error indicators are shown at the top left of the video display if the POST finds an error, and if the system is working enough to give a legible display. If the video is out, these are unseen. But even this short list is sometimes helpful. Much more extensive lists may be obtained.

ERROR CODE	GENERAL FAILURE BLOCK
1xx	System motherboard
100	option configuration error
101	system interrupt circuitry
102	system timer circuitry
103	system timer interrupt
104	system protected mode
105	system 8042 command
106	system converting logic test

107	system NMI test
108	system timer bus test
109	DMA test error
121	unexpected hardware interrupt
131	cassette port error
161	system option error, battery?
162	system option error, run setup
163	time, date not set, run setup
164	memory size error, run setup
2xx	Memory
201	memory test failure
202	memory address error
203	memory address error
3xx	Keyboard
301	keyboard not responding
302	user error or keyboard locked
303	keyboard or system error
304	keyboard error, cmos config error
4xx	Display, mono
401	mono memory, h. sync, or video
408	user indicated attribute error
416	user indicated character set error
424	user indicated 80x25 mode error
432	mono adapter parallel port error
5xx	Display, color
501	color memory, h.sync, or video
508	user indicated attribute error
516	user indicated character set error
524	user indicated 80x25 mode error
532	user indicated 40x25 mode error
540	user indicated 320x200 mode error
548	user indicated 640x200 mode error
556	light pen test
564	user indicated screen paging test
6xx	Diskette drives
601	disk POST error, interface
602	diskette test error
603	diskette size error
606	diskette verify error
607	write protected
608	diskette status returned
610	diskette initialization error
611	timeout

	612	cable or adapter error
	613	bad DMA
	614	DMA boundary error
	621	bad seek
	622	bad CRC
	623	record not found
	624	bad address mark
	625	bad controller seek
	626	data compare error
	627	diskette change line error
	628	diskette removed
	630	A: index stuck high
	631	A: index stuck low
	632	A: track 0 stuck off
	633	A: track 0 stuck on
	640	B: index stuck high
	641	B: index stuck low
	642	B: track 0 stuck off
	643	B: track 0 stuck on
	650	drive speed error
	651	format failure
	652	verify failure
	653	read failure
	654	write failure
	655	controller
	656	drive
	657	write protect stuck protected
	658	change line stuck changed
	659	write protect stuck unprotected
	660	change line stuck unchanged
7xx		Math coprocessor
	702	exception errors test
	703	rounding test
	704	math test 1
	705	math test 2
	706	math test 3
	707	combination test
	708	integer store test
	709	equivalent expressions
	710	exceptions
	711	save state
	712	protected mode test
	713	sensitivity test
9xx		Parallel Printer card

	901	data register latch
	902	control register latch
	903	register address decode
	904	address decode
	910	status line wrap connector
	911	status line bit 8 wrap
	912	status line bit 7 wrap
	913	status line bit 6 wrap
	914	status line bit 5 wrap
	915	status line bit 4 wrap
	916	interrupt wrap
	917	unexpected interrupt
11xx		Com Serial card
	1101	adapter test failure
	1102	card selected feedback
	1103	port 102 register test
	1106	serial option
	1107	com cable
	1108	IRQ3
	1109	IRQ4
	1110	modem status register not clear
	1111	ring indicate
	1112	trailing edge ring indicate
	1113	delta receive line signal detect
	1114	receive line signal detect
	1115	delta receive signal detect
	1116	line control register, bits not set
	1117	line control reg, bits can't be reset
	1118	transmit holding/shift registerstuck
	1119	data ready stuck on
	1120	interrupt enable reg, bits not set
	1121	int enable reg, bits can't be reset
	1122	int pending stuck on
	1123	int ID reg stuck on
	1124	modem control reg bits not set
	1125	modem control reg bits can't be reset
	1126	modem status reg, bits not set
	1127	modem status reg, bits can't be reset
	1128	interrupt ID
	1129	can't force overrun error
	1130	no modem status interrupt
	1131	invalid interrupt pending
	1132	no data ready
	1133	no data available interrupt

Code	Description
1134	no transmit holding interrupt
1135	no interrupts
1136	no received line status interrupt
1137	no receive data available
1138	transmit holding register not empty
1139	no modem status interrupt
1140	transmit holding register not empty
1141	no interrupts
1142	no IRQ4 interrupt
1143	no IRQ3 interrupt
1144	no data transferred
1145	maximum baud rate
1146	minimum baud rate
1148	timeout error
1149	invalid data returned
1150	modem status register error
1151	no DSR and delta DSR
1152	no DSR
1153	no delta DSR
1154	modem status register not clear
1155	no CTS and delta CTS
1156	no CTS
1157	no delta CTS
13xx	Game Control card
1301	adapter failure
1302	joystick test
17xx	Hard drive card
1701	fixed disk or adapter test
1702	time out
1703	drive
1704	controller or drive error
1705	no record found
1706	write fault
1707	track 0 error
1708	head select error
1709	bad ECC
1710	read buffer overrun
1711	bad address mark
1712	undetermined
1713	data compare error
1714	drive not ready
1730	adapter
1731	adapter
1733	adapter

1750	drive verify
1751	drive read
1752	drive write
1753	random read test
1754	drive seek test
1755	controller
1756	controller ECC test
1757	controller head select
1780	drive C: fatal time out
1781	drive D: fatal time out
1782	controller no IPL from hardfile
1790	drive C: non fatal
1791	drive D: non fatal